Foreword by Laura L

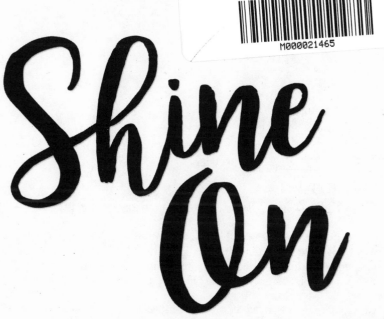

Shine On

The Remarkable True Story
of a Quadruple Amputee

*Sheri
Keep shining
His light!
Matt 5:16
Cyndi Wil~*

Cyndi Desjardins Wilkens

Printed in Canada

ISBN: 978-1-4866-1559-9

Word Alive Press
131 Cordite Road, Winnipeg, MB R3W 1S1
www.wordalivepress.ca

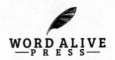
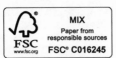

Cataloguing in Publication may be obtained through Library and Archives Canada

For Jesus,

Marc, Cienna, and Liam,
Mom and Dad

I waited patiently for the Lord; He turned to me and heard my cry.
He lifted me out of the slimy pit, out of the mud and mire;
He set my feet on a rock and gave me a firm place to stand.
He put a new song in my mouth, a hymn of praise to our God.

—Psalm 40:1-3

Foreword

If we live long enough, God will give us the opportunity to ask Him, "Why would you let this happen to me?" The experience will be different for each of us, but it will tear us to pieces. Cyndi Desjardins Wilkens found herself in a situation so devastating that my heart wept while reading her story of how she came to the end of herself and found the answers.

I had an overwhelming amount of work on my plate as I sat down to read this book. I wasn't sure how to find the time, and I muttered under my breath that I had to tend to "matters of national importance" that God had put on my heart. I wasn't sure what lesson this little book could teach me that I hadn't already learned through my wealth of painful experiences. Clearly, I had no idea how I would be drawn into this staggering story. I placed everything else aside to read every word, and my attention was captured by the unbelievable circumstances in which Cyndi found herself. After reading Cyndi's story, the difficult chapters in my life paled in comparison. There aren't many women who could say they faced such a challenge as the one Cyndi writes about in this book.

Why would God give any of us more than we think we can handle on a certain day? What is it that we discover in the moments that we think will crush us? These are the questions that will be faced in this book as this precious woman describes a series of events that would break any of us if we had to face them. They broke her. They crushed her. I felt the weight of her pain in every word as I journeyed alongside of her, asking the same question that she was asking of God: "Why?"

It is in the beauty of the unfolding of this story, and the benefit of hindsight, that we see how God weaves a perfect storm into each of our lives to deliver to us a perfect gift at the end of it. Whether you are facing your storm right now or you can relate to a past situation in your own life, you will see God breathe the answers into your soul as you inhale *Shine On*.

Thank you, Cyndi, for writing a most difficult story with a most stunning ending. I found myself undone at the goodness of God, His kindness, His Fatherly heart, and His unfailing love. It brought me back to Hosea 6:1: "*Come, let us return to the Lord. He has torn us to pieces, but he will heal us; he has injured us, but he will bind up our wounds.*"

> *But what can I say? He has spoken to me, and he himself has done this. I will walk humbly all my years because of this anguish of my soul. Lord, by such things people live; and my spirit finds life in them too. You restored me to health and let me live.*
>
> *Surely it was for my benefit that I suffered such anguish. In your love you kept me from the pit of destruction; you have put all my sins behind your back.*

—Isaiah 38:15–17

Laura Lynn Tyler Thompson
Inspirational Speaker
Author of *Relentless Redemption*
TV host of *The 700 Club Canada* and *Laura Lynn and Friends*

Introduction

The lids of my eyes were very heavy. I could see my lashes as they slowly lifted. The light was more than my dry and stinging eyes could bear. Blue eyes stared back at me with a look of compassion and love. But there was something else ... an unfamiliar intensity. My lids wanted to close. I tried to force them open to focus on my husband's face. My heart felt warm, and I was so happy to see the depth of love looking back at me. "Honey, you've been very ill and they've had to amputate ..." His voice cracked. I searched his face, looking for some kind of clue to tell me why I sensed so much pain from him and in me. "... Your hands and feet."

Confusion swirled through my mind as a deep ache gripped my chest—the ache of immense suffering. Pain I had experienced before.

"Honey." His fingers gently touched my cheek as I looked up to see the children's photos hanging from an IV pole above my bed, happy photos of all of us staring back at me with love. My heart was breaking into a million pieces. I longed to hold my children in my arms.

"They have these things called prosthetics." Marc rested his hand on the bed beside my arm. "I've been doing a lot of research ..." He sounded scared, as if trying to convince himself and me at the same time. "We'll get you some. You'll lead a normal life again. We'll get our lives back."

What was he saying? It just couldn't be true. I tried to speak, but no words came. *Please God—let this be a dream.* A sinking, overwhelming feeling crashed down on me as my eyes became heavier and heavier. Darkness threatened to overtake me. *Truly God, haven't we been through enough?*

Part One

It started out as a small, white light.

Immediately I knew who it was and why He was there.

The light felt warm and inviting.

I knew it would welcome me; still, I was afraid.

It was a beautiful light, but I was not ready.

The echo of my voice resonated inside my head.

"Please not now," I cried, hot tears running down my even hotter cheeks.

Images of my children's faces flashed in front of me, play-by-play images of the long journey I had taken to be called "Mama."

"I'm not ready ..."

1

"Let the beloved of the LORD rest secure in him, for he shields him all day long, and the one the LORD loves rests between his shoulders."

—Deuteronomy 33:12

WHEN I WAS A LITTLE GIRL, MY DAD OFTEN TOOK ME FOR LONG WALKS in the forest. Just as we would near the entrance of the trail, he would hold out his hand and I would run to grab it. Sometimes he would let me ride on his shoulders. Calloused fingers wrapped around my hands as he swung me up and onto his strong back. I knew that those hands would not let me fall.

As we walked through the forest, whether it was spring, winter, or fall, we would look for signs of wildlife. My dad had grown up on a 400-acre farm on the east coast of Canada. He had experience trapping his own food, hunting, and fishing because he helped feed his younger siblings when his father left.

Sometimes we would come across the tracks of a small animal, perhaps a squirrel, or we would hear a pheasant running through the brush. Oftentimes we found a small pond and looked for different types of turtles and fish. But once in a while we would find the treasure of a moose or deer track, and Dad would point out the difference.

I didn't get as excited about the wildlife or the tracks as I did about being in the forest. There, surrounded by towering trees, I felt closest to God. It was as if His presence was strongest amongst His great creation. I would turn in a circle, looking up into the sky, the trees around me reaching toward the heavens as though they were praising Him.

Our faith is like a forest. The leaves that fall from the trees can cover it and cause it to be lost or hidden. Or it can be as tall as the tallest tree with many branches representing all the trials we have endured. All those branches reach for the sky, knowing that it is only His strong arms that can carry us through.

❋ ❋ ❋

I was born into trial. It took several days for me to come into this world, as my feet decided they wanted to enter first. In 1968, women were anaesthetized if they needed a C-section; therefore, my mother was not conscious for my delivery.

My father waited to hear that his baby girl had been born. He trained horses at the race track, but he was about to change careers and become a truck driver. My mother was a secretary and had long desired to have a baby girl. She couldn't wait to hold me in her arms.

"Where is my baby?" were the first words she asked when she awoke. But she didn't receive the answer she had hoped for.

The nurse responded abruptly, "There is something wrong with your baby; she has been transferred to Sick Children's Hospital." She then proceeded to tell my mother that I would never speak "properly."

I often think back to how my mother must have felt in that moment. The fear that could have taken her captive. I had been born with a partial cleft palette, a congenital deformation that causes a small opening leading into the canal above the roof of the mouth. A team of plastic surgeons performed several operations. When I was two years old, they inserted a prosthesis. Miraculously, I did not have any speech impediment.

My father transferred jobs frequently and we moved around a lot. I attended many different schools. I learned to make friends fast and hold onto them as long as I could. Although it appeared I was surrounded by chaos and confusion—living in different homes, sometimes even hotels—every night my mother would sit beside the beds of my younger brother and me and show us how to pray. I would kneel down and recite, "Now I lay me down to sleep," a very simple prayer. I would speak to God about my day, thank Him for my blessings, and pray for my hopes and dreams. I would then pray for my family and for the children around the world.

While living in London, Ontario, we attended a Baptist church. It was the longest we had stayed in one area and I loved it there, making many new friends. I would dress up in my very best clothes—a green velvet dress, topped off by white kid gloves and patent leather shoes—and sing "Jesus Loves Me" and "This Little Light of Mine" with great joy in my heart. In Sunday school, I received a little yellow pin embossed with a picture of Jesus. The words "Jesus loves me" circled Him. I treasured that pin and carried it with me as we relocated several more times.

In grade three in West Toronto, I made many more new friends at school. I felt settled and thankful that it looked as though we would be staying for quite some time. We did settle there and I attended high school in the same area.

I developed breasts early and was teased a lot for wearing a bra, as I was one of the first girls in my grade six class to do so. "Round turtle, square turtle, snapping turtle!" the boys would say as they snuck up behind me and pulled my bra strap. I would spend my days holding my shoulders in, praying that the boys would not notice and make fun of me.

When I started high school, I found a way to express myself through writing poetry. My teenage angst was summarized in poems. For the most part I was a good student, but I would sit at the back of the class, feet tapping against one another while I wrote a poem, hoping the teacher wouldn't notice that I wasn't paying attention. I had a few close friends by that time, and I would show them my works, passing them back and forth during class. There was a poem for every crush, heartbreak, loss, and all the confusion I faced as a teenager. I was very shy and afraid to talk to boys. I didn't know how to interact with them. I had no confidence and low self-esteem. I mostly bowed my head as I made my way through the high school hallways, trying to get up the courage to say hi.

Then I discovered theatre. My parents saw my passion and put me into extracurricular theatre and television acting classes. My self-confidence started to rise. I was still extremely shy around boys, but I had found another outlet. All my daydreams centred on studying acting in New York or Los Angeles.

When I graduated from high school, I started saving every penny to achieve this goal. After many yard sales, and working full and part-time jobs, I had amassed sufficient funds to live and attend a program in Pasadena, California.

I was in my mid-twenties, and an older student than most, but I was thankful to be doing what I loved—studying theatre. I purchased a bicycle and would bike to school up a very large mountain and back down again. I met people from all over the United States and truly loved my independence, but I missed my family. At the end of the program, I knew it was time to go home.

I returned to Toronto and obtained a full-time position with a pharmaceutical company as a sales secretary. I was twenty-seven and living in an affluent area of the city on my own. I found myself surrounded by very close friends I had met through work and life. I launched my own theatre production company with one of them. We produced and directed plays and ran one at a local theatre. We rehearsed wherever we could—in school classrooms, parks, and at each other's houses.

For my twenty-ninth birthday, one of my best friends, Michelle, purchased tickets to a rock concert. As I was getting ready to go, applying lipstick in the mirror in the small bathroom of my tiny one-bedroom apartment, she mentioned that a group of people was coming from her work.

When we arrived at the concert at Maple Leaf Gardens in Toronto, we took our seats and waited for the rest of the group to join us. We were joined by two young men, and one in particular caught my eye. He was introduced to me as Marc.

In many ways, I was still like that shy little girl in high school, but we went to a diner after the show and I listened to Marc speak about his family, weaving stories to bring them to life as if he were an expert storyteller. As I had grown up with storytellers, that appealed to me.

My mother, and my grandmother before her, would tell me stories of their childhoods as we drove on long car trips each summer. My favourite story was one of my grandmother's, the Salvation Army tale. My grandmother and her eleven siblings lived in an old century home on the east coast of Canada. They waited patiently all week for Saturday night when their mom and dad would go out to dinner and dancing. As soon as their parents were out the door, they grabbed large pots and wooden spoons. They would create their own instruments, and they became the Salvation

Army band, playing songs and singing at the top of their lungs. All evening they danced around the house and even on the table, entertaining one another and then quickly putting everything back in its proper place before their parents returned.

Marc's story rivalled this one. He told a story of his father surviving the fury of an angry bull and trying to outrun him. The kindness and warmth in his blue eyes intrigued me. I wanted to get to know him more.

Michelle and I took a cab back to my apartment. In the backseat, I turned to her and said, "Now, if he were to ask me for coffee, I would accept."

She looked at me skeptically. She had tried to set me up with many of her friends from work without success.

When I returned home that night, I could not stop thinking about the warm blue eyes that had looked at me across the table, or the stories Marc had told. I didn't know whether or not Michelle would take me seriously and suggest to him that we go for coffee. As I drifted off to sleep, I told myself that if it was meant to be she would. Several weeks went by and I heard nothing.

Then one evening, as I was driving home from a sales meeting in Niagara Falls, my phone rang. I answered to hear Michelle's voice on the other line. "I spoke to Marc, and I have his phone number for you. He said you could give him a call any time." My heart raced with excitement ... but had I heard her correctly? *I* was going to call *him*? I thought she would arrange for him to call me, not have me call him! I spent the two-hour drive home trying to imagine how I was going to do this.

I may have let a few days go by, far too afraid to pick up the phone, but somehow I finally managed to take a deep breath and dial his number. We spent a bit of time on the phone and arranged to meet one evening after my part-time job at a bridal shop where I sold wedding gowns to supplement my income. The girls at the shop and I had become very good friends, and they cheered me on as I left to go on my big date.

Marc lived in an apartment building in an area called Yonge and Eglinton in another unique part of downtown Toronto. I was very nervous as I walked into the lobby of the building and pushed the button to let him know I was there. He came down and took me to a local restaurant where we spoke about our lives and shared our hopes and dreams into the early hours of the morning. As he walked me to my car, we shared our first kiss.

This compassionate and kind man came from such a chaotic childhood. As I grew to know him more, something deep inside told me I would marry him.

When we first started dating, we agreed to drive to Nova Scotia for a vacation and for him to meet some of my family. I was excited to show him the province where I had spent part of my childhood, and of which I had very fond memories.

We stood on the deck of a ferry crossing the Bay of Fundy. The wind was blowing through my hair as I looked into his blue eyes.

"So, when are you going to tell me you love me?" I asked. I had no idea how those words came out of my mouth. It was as if somebody else was speaking. We had only been together for a few months.

His eyes widened. "Are you so sure already?"

I looked at him and smiled confidently as I nodded. "Aren't you?"

A year and a half later, on Christmas Eve, Marc took me to dinner at a restaurant and with shaking hands proposed to me, and I accepted.

I poured all of myself into our wedding planning. We were married in a 150-year-old church on Lake Simcoe. My father drove us to the church in his 1968 Cadillac convertible.

We were blessed with an incredibly beautiful wedding day. After weeks of rain, the sun broke through that morning. Both of my parents walked me down the aisle. When I looked up at Marc, tears were streaming down his face. Surrounded by our friends and family, I had never felt enveloped in so much joy and love, so hopeful for the future.

2

"He reached down from on high and took hold of me; he drew me out of deep waters."

—Psalm 18:16

When I was a little girl, I prayed to God every night. I would imagine myself walking up a tall stairway to heaven. At the top of the stairs, on a little platform amongst the stars, I would meet God. I never saw His face, but I looked at Him with childlike wonder, feeling His presence. I would kneel down on the platform with my teddy bear in my arms, and my nightgown falling around me in a pool of fabric. I would tell Him about my day and share with Him my hopes and dreams. It is easy to speak to God when you see Him as love with arms wide open, ready to embrace you.

I sighed heavily as I looked at my reflection in the mirror. *Where is that little girl now?*

Marc and I had been married over three years, and it had not been easy. In fact, I never imagined that life could be so full of pain. Hope seemed far and unreachable. My childhood had been idyllic compared to this. How many times over the last years had I wondered if, by marrying my husband, I had also taken on his life cycle? It was as though on the day we married, he arrived with his bags packed full of childhood trauma that made it difficult for him to break through or feel joy. The pain in my heart was as overwhelming as a runaway train on which I was trapped and unable to escape.

I did what I always do when I feel the world collapsing in on me. I ran a hot bath—so hot that it felt as though it was on the edge of boiling. What was it about a hot bath that always soothed my soul? Perhaps it was the vulnerability of being exposed, or the time it gave me to think, to question God, to wait for Him to answer.

As I slid my weary, broken spirit into the bathtub, it occurred to me that I had hit rock bottom. Those silly but powerful words made me think of somebody passed out on a dirty motel room floor, coming around to the realization that they had lost everything—money, family, and, most importantly, hope.

The darkness was closing in on me, and I didn't know what to do. I felt as though I could not possibly pick myself up and carry on. I looked at the ceiling, imagining, through my tears, that it was a gateway to God, and I begged Him to carry me, for surely I could no longer carry myself.

The amount of water seemed to represent the tears I had cried in the first years of our marriage. I lay there with tears rolling down my face, thinking over the past few years and trying to figure out how I had arrived at this place of lost hope.

Just before we were married, I had accepted a new position as Marketing Communications Specialist for a Canadian electrical manufacturing company located in Toronto. This role required a very large learning curve, as I would be promoting electrical products with no engineering background. I dedicated countless evenings to studying specifications and coming to understand the products that I would be promoting. I spent many late nights at the office taking on the new challenges I was given, attempting to prove myself. I spent my days immersed in office politics, with no experience. Often I would be the only woman fighting for success amongst men; most days I felt as though I had failed.

Since our wedding, Marc's mother had shown signs of illness. Before long, she was diagnosed with terminal cirrhosis of the liver and hepatitis C. It was likely that we would lose her over the next several months. As she struggled with her addiction to alcohol, we did our best to support her in her suffering. I watched my husband's heart suffering with his mama's.

We had been trying to conceive for a while. All of our friends were starting their families, but month by month we were disappointed. After two years of marriage, we found ourselves sitting side by side in front of a specialist, desperate to hear that he could help us have a baby. In my naivety, I was optimistic that he would be able to solve all our problems. I was ready and anxious to start fertility drugs or whatever it took to become a mother. The papers spread out in front of him like a fan—test results on blood and semen— represented our hopes and dreams. The doctor studied them for a moment before looking up. "You will need a test-tube baby. Save $15,000 and come back and see me then."

I screamed inside my head. *What is that? Why do I need one?* I had been a good girl all my life. Was I being punished for something?

We stood outside the doctor's office as Marc put his arms around me and said, "We will get through this; don't worry, honey." But his words seemed so hollow. *How can he be so matter-of-fact? Why didn't he appear to be as crushed as I was?*

My friends continued to conceive. I put on a happy face and told them how thrilled I was while my heart started to die. I plummeted into a depression. Saving that much money seemed impossible. Then, as if we could take another hit, Marc lost his job. His mother was dying. We needed $15,000 to attempt to have a child. My longing to be a mother already seemed an unreachable dream, and now my husband was jobless. It seemed as though our friends lived idyllic lives as we suffered through one trial after another.

Marc had become a different person. In survival mode, his walls went up and became like a fortress. I was unable to break through, and I could not understand why he didn't feel the loss and pain that I felt. At night, while he struggled to come to terms with the loss of his mother, I floated around in the dark cellar of my own loss. I would reach for his hand, longing for comfort that he could not provide. My marriage started to fall apart. I was alone and afraid. Feelings of isolation and loneliness set in and seared my soul.

That day had been a particularly difficult one. I had spent my lunch break crying on the couch in the bathroom at work, something that was becoming more and more frequent. Cindy and Maria—my confidants—held my hands. One of my coworkers had just brought her baby in for everyone to hold. I glanced at the two of them as I walked by, once again stifling the ache in my heart. I was afraid that if I held that baby in my arms I would not be able to stop the tears, that they would continue for days.

Why me? Lying in the bathtub, I contemplated the blue circles that surrounded me. Marc had meticulously painted them by hand. "Honey," he said as he waved his arm around the room, "I made our bathroom look like an ocean oasis."

I longed for Marc to come in and wipe my tears away, but he was absent. Did he even know how much I was suffering?

I wanted an end to this pain. How could I continue through every day like this— pretending I had a great life, a perfect marriage, and that I didn't desire to be a mom? I was drowning in loss.

I could end it all. It would be so simple … This wasn't the first time I had thought of it. A simple slit to the wrist, and the blood would flow away, and so would the pain. This ache of hopelessness plagued me. I wanted to be rid of it.

A wave of shame overtook me for having such a thought. *How can I even consider hurting God or my parents that way?* I wandered around, lost and confused, in my thoughts and emotions bred of isolation.

I took a long, deep breath. I imagined stretching my arms far into the sky, reaching for God. I could almost feel Him picking me up, placing my feet upon the furry rug on the floor, and carrying me off to bed.

3

"Because of the LORD's great love we are not consumed, for his compassions never fail. They are new every morning; great is your faithfulness."

—Lamentations 3:22-23

My family spent many of our summers on the east coast of Canada. Upon our arrival, my parents would take me to a beach covered in large rocks. Before taking a step to the edge of the water, I would stand and listen to the waves roll in, tasting the salt on my lips.

As I walked across the rocks, my feet would become entangled in washed-up seaweed. It seemed like a long hike to the water, but when I finally arrived the salt water would wash up my legs and spray my face. I loved the ocean, the smell of the air as the salt hit my tongue, the soothing sound of the waves.

Now I lounged on a beach next to a much warmer ocean in the Caribbean. Once again, I could taste the salt on my lips as I listened to the waves rolling in. Beside me, Marc was reading a book. We had arrived a few days ago.

For several months, I had been trying to reach out to him, to breach the fortress that had gone up when we lost his mother. I longed to share with him the thoughts and feelings that had been on my heart.

The fortress walls only thickened through our struggle to have children. The two of us did not mourn the loss of fertility in the same way. In fact, I questioned if he mourned it at all. I had to fight down the anger that I felt, the loneliness that came in the middle of the night, stealthy and ready to attack. I wasn't just lonely because I wanted children. I also struggled with the aching feeling of being alone in my desire for them. I hoped I was wrong.

A few months ago, the phone had rung as I arrived home from work. I prayed these were the results I had been waiting for.

"Ms. Desjardins?" The female voice on the other end line sent my heart racing.

"Yes!" My voice was breathless. I was ready for them to tell me when to come in for insemination.

"I'm afraid we have to cancel your session. You have developed cysts on your ovaries. We cannot proceed from here. But ..." she continued through the lingering silence on my end, "... you can take a break and we can start again in the new year."

I fumbled to hang up the phone before sinking down on the edge of the bed, trying to process what I had just heard. It couldn't be true. I really believed that I was going to be a mother. How many more baby showers would I have to endure? Sobs wracked my body. I felt empty. I had no idea where to turn. I had few friends or family who understood.

I was determined to be a mom, so once again I picked myself up and kept going. Surely God would answer my prayer somehow, some way.

"When do you want to try IVF again?" I would ask Marc.

He would always respond, curtly, "When we have the money."

I started to wonder if he really wanted to have children. Those doubts changed something in me. I started questioning if I could go through another procedure and disappointment.

Now, as he lay beside me on the beach, I wondered how I would tell him what was on my heart.

"I've been thinking," I treaded lightly, knowing how sensitive the topic was, "I don't think I could go through another IVF attempt and be disappointed again." Not waiting for his reaction, I pressed on, part of me afraid he would say he didn't want children at all. "I think I would like to adopt." I bit my lip. How would he react to that idea? I couldn't read his expression. "It would mean that the child would have no genetic parts of us, but I would be okay with that. Would you?"

I held my breath ... waiting for hope to return.

He smiled. That smile made me feel warm and loved deep in my soul.

"I would love any child that belonged to us. It doesn't have to come from us."

I released a sigh so full of relief I thought I might float away.

"God will send us the right child," he said as he leaned over and kissed me.

4

"Surely your goodness and love will follow me all the days of my life, and I will dwell in the house of the LORD forever."

—Psalm 23:6

I WALKED DOWN A HALLWAY WITH A VERY BIG WINDOW AT THE END OF IT. I moved closer, trying to see through the window, but the light shining through it was far too bright. It shone radiantly, in sparkling streams, down upon a beautiful baby girl in a white dress lying on the bed below. Deep within me, and in every part of me, I knew she was my daughter. I reached down and picked her up, holding her close to my heart. The longing and pain subsided. The joy in my heart, the feeling of completeness, could only come from being a mother.

My eyes flew open. Was this a vision or a dream? Could God send me a baby? I didn't want to get out of bed. I wanted to take a moment to bask in the feeling of holding a child in my arms. It was a feeling of great joy, hope, and love. When hope bubbles in your heart, it is easy to have faith. That faith motivated me to push forward with our home study as part of the adoption process. I prayed for God to send me that little girl.

We listed our profile on an adoption website. By day I held the secret in my heart, and at night I fielded phone calls, screening birth mothers as they screened me.

Early on I received a call from a young woman in the United States who was three months pregnant. The first time she called we spent a few hours on the phone. When I hung up, I walked down the stairs of our two-story home and into the living room where Marc was sitting, watching television.

"I think this might be the one." I proceeded to tell him all about her.

"She's only three months pregnant?" he asked. I knew what he was thinking. It was too early to be hopeful; anything could happen in the next six months. He was right, but that hope continued bubbling in my heart. We had shared such a wonderful connection over the phone. As we continued our telephone conversations, she confirmed that she was not only choosing us to be the baby's parents, but adamant that she was not going to change her mind. Every time fear and worry seeped in, she seemed to understand instinctively how I felt, and would reinforce that she was choosing us to be the baby's parents and could not be swayed.

A few months later we flew to Florida over a weekend to meet with our birth mother. As we walked up to the desk of our hotel, we were greeted with a warmer-than-usual welcome.

The receptionist's name, according to her nametag, was *Rita.* I thought perhaps that was a good sign, as it was also my grandmother's name.

"What brings you to our city?"

Marc blurted out, "We're here to meet a potential birth mother."

I stared at him, shocked. It was very out of character for him to be telling this to a stranger.

Her smile reflected in her eyes as she proceeded to tell us she had three adopted children and was about to adopt a set of twins from Bulgaria.

Anticipation running high, we changed our clothing from the long flight and headed to a local restaurant to meet the woman who carried our hopes and dreams. As we walked through the lobby, Rita cheered us on.

We had to wait for some time, and each moment made me more and more nervous. My stomach was churning and panic started to creep in. The restaurant seemed to be getting busier and the noise louder.

Time dragged on until I noticed a young girl sitting on a bench at the front of the restaurant. She had long, brown hair and she was wearing a white maternity top. Was that her?

As I walked over, my eyes met her brown ones, so similar to mine. She straightened on the bench. "Cyndi?"

My heart raced and danced all at once. I nodded, a smile crossing my face. We went to join Marc at the table. As we sat and talked, I ached to reach out and touch her belly, to tell the baby how much I loved her.

We spent the day together, first at the restaurant and then at the hotel pool, talking about our lives, our families, and our hopes for the baby.

Eventually, the birth mother went home, and Marc and I walked back through the hotel hand-in-hand.

"So?" Rita inquired.

We both looked up and said, "She is the one." We were ecstatic.

On our flight home, we started picking out names.

※ ※ ※

A few days later, I received the anticipated call from the woman I had come to think of as our angel.

"I had my ultrasound, and I have news." I held my breath, waiting. "It's a baby girl."

Tears and joy came all at once. A girl. Just like in my vision. I hoped that my daughter and I would be best friends, just as my mom and I were. The baby could arrive within the next month, and I had barely been sleeping in my anxiousness and excitement.

"I have to call Marc right away," I shared with her.

I knew my husband would be sitting in his cubicle, waiting for the call. He worked in a technology office, and all his coworkers were eagerly following our quest to adopt.

He told me later that, as soon as he heard the news, he stood up. "It's a girl!" he announced. I could hear his coworkers cheering.

Although it seemed like an endless period of waiting, it was no time before we were sitting on an airplane on our way to Florida.

"This is it," Marc said as he held my hand. At our birth mother's request, the hospital would induce her so that we could be present for the delivery of our baby girl.

As I sat on the airplane looking down at the clouds, I couldn't help but reflect on the events that had led us here. So much pain and sadness at first, then came the hope of adoption. Any child could be a child of mine, as Marc had said. No matter where she came from, if she was ours, we would love her. I was going to be a mom. *Please God, don't let her back out.*

For five years I had waited to be a mom. I had dreamt about many moments with great anticipation: changing diapers, the first moment I would hold the baby in my arms, the first bottle, and the first word, "Mama." And, of course, finally parking in that one spot in the parking lot labelled, *New Mom*.

What would it be like in the delivery room? Our angel had asked if I would like to cut the cord, and I had immediately agreed.

I imagined them placing our baby in a little crib, proudly displaying the name we had chosen and wheeling her into the room with us. I wiped the tears from my eyes as we prepared for landing.

❊ ❊ ❊

That night we had dinner with our angel and then went back to our hotel to once again share our hopes.

"I have a gift for you." She handed me a beautifully wrapped gift bag.

I opened the package to find a Willow Tree figurine of a husband and wife holding a tiny baby. I discreetly studied our birth mother, marvelling at her strength. But would she be able to stay strong and place this baby in our arms?

"I just know you will make great parents," she assured us. Where did her courage come from?

I was even more inspired the next day as I watched her labour for several hours. Then it was time.

Marc stood near our angel's head and held her hand as I coached her.

"Come," said the doctor, "put your hands here." I placed them where she suggested, waiting with anticipation for the baby to come out. Before I knew it, the doctor was holding the baby out to me. "It's time to cut the cord!" A specialized instrument was thrust into my hands.

I took a breath and gazed at our angel. She had just given birth to our child. She had just given us the most beautiful gift one could receive.

The nurses set the baby on the table, with heat lamps above her.

She hasn't cried yet. Panic gripped my heart.

Please God, let her cry, I begged silently. I felt as though the entire room was silent, waiting for a sound. Then it came. The most beautiful, piercing cry of our baby. I couldn't see through my own tears, but I sensed tears in the eyes of everyone in the room.

I walked over to see our little girl's beautiful face. When I reached out, she wrapped her tiny baby fingers around my pinky. Marc and I were still crying as I whispered, "Cienna, I get to be your mama, and I will never leave your side."

Our beautiful birth mother spent some time in the room saying goodbye to the little angel she had the courage to place in our arms. Time seemed to tick by very slowly as we waited in the nursery. I could tell by his pacing and fidgeting that Marc was concerned and scared. Eventually the door opened and a nurse walked across the room to place our beautiful baby, wrapped in blankets, into my arms. I gazed down at her little face. We had been through so much pain and suffering, but in that moment the heartache evaporated.

The nurse slid a card into the holder attached to the crib. I hurried over, expecting the name we had chosen to be displayed. A moment I had dreamed of.

But in place of the name, I saw only the letters BUFA.

"Her name is Cienna, not BUFA." I cocked my head as I looked at the nurse.

"Oh, that stands for Baby Up For Adoption," she replied frankly. She explained that BUFA would remain until the legal waiting period had passed and they knew that our birth mother would not change her mind. "The baby will stay in the nursery until that time," she added.

In this state, that was two days. I was frantic. Would they prevent us from being with her? Now that she was in my arms, I couldn't let her go. "But our birth mother told you she won't change her mind," I argued. The nurse left to investigate while I held our baby and gave her a bottle.

Later the nurse returned. "Well, your birth mother is adamant that she will not change her mind and has threatened to bring all of you into the room with her if we don't allow you to be with the baby." My chest tightened. That would be awkward and difficult for everyone. The nurse must have realized that too. She sighed. "We'll get you a hospital room so you can be with the baby."

I studied Cienna's face as she drank happily from the bottle. A shiver of delight rippled through me. I was holding my little girl in my arms, and I would never let her go.

We stayed with our baby girl at the hospital for two days while her birth mom recuperated. The hospital provided a special dinner for all new moms and fathers. Our angel asked me to join her for this steak dinner. Marc remained in the room, lovingly caring for Cienna as her birth mother and I sat across from one another and planned our daughter's future.

"I think she will be very independent," she told me as they placed the food before us.

We both agreed she would be independent, headstrong, and beautiful.

"Please raise her in the gospel," she asked, and I promised I would.

Returning to Canada with our new baby proved to be much more complicated than expected. We spent nights in our hotel room in Florida with Marc diligently filling out paperwork as I fed her and held her in my arms. After four days, we travelled to New York State, where we waited for her passport to arrive. When it did, we would be able to cross the border and enter Canada. Then, we could take her home.

Marc was expected to return to work, so my mom joined me to help me take care of Cienna in a motel room near the border. Five days later her passport arrived and I called Marc. "Come and get us; we are coming home!" I cried in joy.

After a long drive, we carried Cienna into her new bedroom and placed her on the change table. With help from friends—the same friends who had held my hands as I cried in the bathroom at work—we had painted the room with big white clouds on a blue-sky background and made wispy yellow curtains that floated on the breeze drifting through the window. Our tiny girl looked around, her little eyes appearing to take everything in, and, as though she felt the love that we poured upon her, she smiled.

A few moments later, I was changing her diaper and called Marc over. I picked her up and set her on my chest, pointing out a small birthmark on her back. His eyes widening, he reached out and gently traced it with his finger. "She has the same birthmark as you."

My heart raced with excitement. "I noticed it in the hotel room and couldn't wait to show you. It's in the exact same spot as mine. It's as if God was giving his stamp of approval."

Marc wrapped his arms around me. "She was made to be ours, and this is His kiss."

I felt as though I could float away on the feeling of joy. We were a family, at last.

Every morning I brought the baby downstairs with me and settled her in her little chair while I prepared food for the day. One morning I was stirring a pot of oatmeal for breakfast, and Cienna was cooing and chatting with happy baby noises. My heart filled. *I could easily fill my house with children.* I loved being a mom.

But Marc had no desire to grow our family … yet. He adored his little girl, but was concerned about the debt we had taken on in adopting her, so after I returned to work, we sold our house and moved one hour north of the city into a house with a smaller mortgage.

The small suburb we moved to—nestled between two larger cities—had a population of approximately two thousand. The area that we were in was a thirty-year-old development with large, ranch-style homes sprawled upon wide lots. Each home was surrounded by several tall trees that reached for the skies and offered shade for the small hiking trails meandering between them. Our lot was situated on a main street, surrounded by peach and apple trees. It had more gardens than I thought a working mom could possibly manage. It didn't take long for us to settle into the community and make many new friends.

As Cienna grew and the years went by, we spent many sun-kissed summer hours in the backyard. The branches of the peach trees bowed low, heavy with peaches. I spent weekends making jams and jellies from all the berries growing in the gardens.

I continued commuting to work, and my new position required quite a bit of travel across North America. I now reported directly to the CEO of the company. My responsibilities included leading and motivating our sales and product development teams. Although the position carried great stress at times, it also offered me many opportunities to grow.

The weekends were spent making cupcakes, dancing around the house and yard, and playing with my little dream girl. She was my world.

5

"For great is his love toward us, and the faithfulness of the LORD endures forever."

—Psalm 117:2

SOMETHING DEEP DOWN INSIDE OF ME WAS TRYING TO BREAK FREE, BUT the brick wall that held it in there was a stronghold in my heart.

At night, and even in the very few quiet moments of the day, whispers tried to surface. But I pushed them back into that stronghold. They couldn't be true.

I wasn't feeling very well. Marc had been travelling a lot lately, and I was very run down. One day while driving in the car, he pulled over and turned to face me, his hands shaking. "Honey, there's something I have to tell you."

The whispers pushed hard at the stronghold door as my stomach flipped over and over. I held my breath, knowing what he was going to say. I was overcome by a surge of nausea mixed with waves of deep sadness.

"I've been unfaithful." His voice trembled when he said the words I'd long been dreading.

My ears rang as the whispers broke free of the dark cellar in which I had locked them away. I felt completely exposed.

"I'm so sorry, and I understand if you want me to leave." His chin dropped to his chest and he began to sob.

Anger brewed up inside of me.

"Is it someone I know? Do you love her?" A burning shame grew stronger in my chest. I took a deep breath and exhaled as if to release the pain. I hoped it wasn't someone permanent.

"No, it was just once when I was travelling." He lifted his head. His hands steadied and he locked his eyes on mine. "It was so easy; I figured no one would know. I've made a terrible mistake." His blue eyes reflected deep regret. "I've hurt you and our little girl." Tears still streamed down his cheeks. "I am so sorry."

The humiliation that washed over me was powerfully effective at making me feel used and dumb.

"I'll need to think about it all." I sighed, turning away from his gaze. *How could he?*

Through the course of the day, the whispers became loud voices. Voices that screamed anger, hate, and "why."

What would it be like to raise our daughter by myself?

I wanted my life back. I wanted my marriage back. I wanted more children. We were in the process of looking at adopting another child. My dreams seemed shattered once again.

Dreams I had clung to for so long.

❋ ❋ ❋

As I drove to work the next day, I tried to see through the tears in my eyes and the heavy rain on the windshield. My mind went over the special moments Marc and I had shared. On our first date, he had opened up and shared the story of his tumultuous childhood with me.

"I was born in Germany. We moved here when I was two years old with my older brother and sister. We lived a very comfortable life. My father used to be a veterinarian and farmer, but when I was five years old his business partner passed away and his children severed the relationship. We had to walk away from it all and move."

He had heard his father and mother speaking about leaving. Where would they go? What about his friends? He knelt down and silently, in his head, he prayed. He had heard God spoken of before. Where had it been? Not from his parents; they didn't believe in God, and he had never been to a church. *Dear God, I don't know if you're up there, or if you even exist, but if you do, please make this stop. Please make it all okay.*

He wiped the tears from his face as he stood up again. He wasn't sure if he had done it right, but he hoped God had heard him.

Within a matter of a few weeks, their things were packed in the back of the car. As they drove away, Marc looked out the back window at the words he had scrawled in the snow: *Bye Jeff*. Jeff was his best friend, and he didn't even have a chance to say goodbye.

They moved across the country, and over the next few years lived in various homes across Canada. Just as they would get settled and Marc would start making friends, they would pack up and leave. He grew accustomed to having a sick and uneasy feeling in his stomach on a regular basis.

After settling in Northern Ontario, the family started to feel secure again when his father found a farming venture with a new partner. However, as Marc described it, "After a year, the partner embezzled money and fled the country. My dad was held legally responsible, and as we watched everything taken away, we fled to the Dominican Republic. I never felt normal there. Everything was so different; I felt out of place."

Marc's father took care of a farm for an affluent businessman, performing veterinary-like tasks. One day there was quite a commotion on the farm. One of the workers accidentally cut his leg with a chainsaw. The gash ran deep into an artery on his right thigh. "The man was hysterical, and if my father hadn't been there, the man would have died." Marc explained that his father had knocked the man out and sewn him up with the supplies in his veterinary kit. As he spoke, I could see love for his dad shining through. The same way it had the day we first met.

Soon afterwards, chaos re-entered their lives. Marc's father was thrown into jail in Santo Domingo for an unknown reason. He had to pay an astronomical fine, and the family was deported with one-way tickets to Puerto Rico. "From there, we went to the United States, driving around in an old clunker of a car while Papa tried to find employment."

He found a position on a farm in New York State. They had been comfortably living there for a year when the authorities showed up at the door and took away his mother. She was gone for two weeks when they came and took his father as well. As the older sibling, Marc's brother became the caregiver.

When his mother returned a few weeks later, she said they were moving once again. This time their father was being extradited to Canada, where he would be incarcerated. They moved into a small town in Northern Ontario and rented a small apartment above a flower shop.

They were starting fresh once again, and this time they were determined to make it work. For a while, no one knew about his father. His mom told Marc to tell people that his parents were separated. But then news about his dad made it to local paper, and Marc was confronted at school and teased about his father being in jail.

The years passed, and Marc started making more friends. His teenage years were spent partying with friends, drinking heavily, and abusing drugs. His feelings of unsettlement and constant insecurity did not go away. They haunted him well into his college years.

His mother helped him prepare for college, where he studied business management and marketing and found his career path in computer technology. Not long after graduation, he accepted an inside sales position at a computer company in the city. Eventually he began working for a technology distribution company, which led him to meeting me.

※ ※ ※

I sat in the parking lot at work, unable to summon the strength to go in. The memories of our life together, our love, combined with my tears, had exhausted me.

I knew even before he said the words that I would forgive him. Perhaps it was something in the way I was raised. Perhaps it was because, selfishly, I didn't want to walk away from everything we could have. The life I expected us to have. I would not give up on him. Residing in the dark recesses of my heart was a place that held onto faith. I knew that God would give me the man that Marc was going to be.

6

"The seed that fell among the thorns represents others who hear God's word, but all too quickly the message is crowded out by the worries of this life, the lure of wealth, and the desire for other things, so no fruit is produced."

—Mark 4:18-19, NLT

DEEP IN THE FOREST, BEFORE THE ARRIVAL OF SPRING, THE SUN CAN shine warm enough to start the melting of snow. As a result of the melting snow, water trickles down through streams, waterways, and into the ground. A slow melt in the forest can take several months. It's a time of anticipation, when only the trees can hear the sounds of melting snow falling down upon the ground, or the trickling of water.

There is much more going on under the earth as the seeds wait patiently to grow. All are waiting anxiously for the sun. Waiting to shine in all their splendour, bringing joy to all who see them and glory to their creator.

Does a hardened heart melt in a similar way? Slowly, as it is exposed moment-by-moment, day-by-day to the light? My heart was becoming hard.

What can cause a hardened heart? The moment I heard of Marc's infidelity, I hardened mine. Vengeance festered like a tumour, and although I had no heart to cheat on Marc, I found other ways to be unfaithful. I took another lover. This lover gave the false impression of filling me up, but I wanted more. This lover was purely of flesh. For every cold slight and fortress wall that went up from my husband, I found reason to hit his insecurities where it would wound him the most. I went shopping and charged everything to my credit card.

The journey to a hardened heart usually ends with an unfaithful one, and I was carrying the signs of an unfaithful heart. I envied what others had. My desires became a swimming pool in the backyard, perhaps a second property. I told myself people would see me differently if I owned all these things. I would have a happier, more fulfilled life, so I worked hard to achieve that extra bonus or rise in stature.

Some days there was a little gnaw at my heart that said, *What happened to that little girl who loved me so? Why have you left me?*

But desire can be a lonely companion. I tried to fill the emptiness inside me without searching to find where it came from. If I had just searched my heart to see why I felt so empty, I may have turned back to Him.

❊ ❊ ❊

I wanted desperately to build our family, and I put increasing pressure on Marc. Although a few years had passed, and I appeared to have forgiven him, our marriage was invisibly strained.

We tried adopting, and attempt after attempt failed. Each new try brought excitement and then disappointment. We decided to try adopting from Africa and handed in our paperwork, then waited anxiously to hear that we had been put on the long waiting list. However, within a matter of days, we found out that the company we had chosen to adopt from had gone bankrupt.

We felt confident enough to sit in front of the specialist once again and ask about in vitro. This time we resigned ourselves to whatever answer would come. Perhaps we were to be a three-person family.

"We are very realistic in coming here. If you tell us that we can't have any more children, well … we will go buy a hot tub and get on with our lives," Marc said, and we all laughed.

The doctor surprised us both and recommended a specialized program in Argentina. We agreed that we should give it a try. We had friends in Argentina, which made travelling to a foreign country seem so much easier.

"We could make it our tenth wedding anniversary celebration," Marc suggested.

Our trip was filled with romantic dinners and special times spent with friends. We came home pregnant. For the first time in my life, I took a test and it was positive.

Although there were some complications, my pregnancy was relatively easy, and before long Marc was holding our baby boy in his arms with a smile of fatherly pride on his face. During my delivery, I felt such closeness to Marc, as he didn't leave my side.

At Cienna's birth, I had been the first to hold her. Now I lay there watching Marc pass the baby to my mom, who had also been in the room with us.

"We have travelled the Western hemisphere to build our family," Marc joked.

I looked into my baby boy's eyes. *Perhaps this is it; no more trials. We have accomplished our goal and we can settle down and enjoy life as a happy family.*

For the first time in a very long time, I felt complete.

7

"And we know that in all things God works for the good
of those who love him, who have been called according
to his purpose."

—Romans 8:28

OUR THREE-MONTH-OLD BABY BOY, LIAM, HAD THE CROUP AGAIN. I WAS
sure of it and prepared to take him to the hospital for the second time for
the specially-administered medication.

He didn't like car rides and screamed all the way there. My mom accompanied me and she tried to be reassuring, but I was frustrated.

As I drove the SUV along the tree-lined side streets, I tried to recall
when the first time was that he had the croup. I was sure it was just a few
short weeks ago.

Liam did not like to be put down to sleep alone. It wasn't long before
I realized I would have to temporarily move into his room with him, as he
woke up so many times during the night. When he did, I would pick him
up and settle him on the bed beside me.

The first trip to the hospital had been relatively easy. It seemed as
though we didn't have to wait very long before the respiratory therapist
came in and gave him the mask he needed. I carried him out and within a
few hours he started to show signs of improvement.

On this return trip, I turned into the emergency parking lot, hoping
there wouldn't be a long wait. My heart dropped when I saw the parking
lot was full.

I gripped the steering wheel. "We'll have to find other parking." The
frustration I'd felt earlier was turning to anger. I was angry at the hospital
for not having ample parking. I was angry that I was back here again. I was

very angry with Marc, as it seemed I was always the one taking the children to the hospital. I longed for him to be with me. Then I looked in the rear-view mirror at my little boy, crying and screaming. In spite of the circumstances, I smiled, thinking back to the first time we'd come to the hospital. He'd cried all the way to the hospital that time too. When we arrived, I set him, still secured in his car seat, up on the desk at the nursing triage station. The nurse reached out and removed his little booties to touch his bare toes. As soon he saw her pretty eyes he stopped crying. He smiled and cooed and flashed his very, very long eyelashes at her.

I looked down at him and chuckled. "He will be a heart breaker."

After a long search for parking we found a spot. It was snowy and cold out, and I chose to make the extra-long trek through the hospital corridors instead of walking outside in the blistering cold. It seemed to take forever, but we finally entered the doors to the emergency area. My fears had been well-founded. This time there was a very long line.

After waiting for what felt like hours, we were put into a curtained cubicle where we sat and waited some more, this time for a doctor to arrive. The man next to me was coughing profusely and swearing at the hospital for taking so long to see him.

"I do hope he stops all that coughing," my mom said. "I'm concerned we're all going to catch what he has."

"He should be nicer to the doctors here." I pulled Liam closer to my chest. "I'm sure they're doing their best."

After several more hours, a doctor finally came in and administered the medication. I carried my baby boy out in his little baby bucket back down the extensive hallways to the car.

When I finally went to bed, I had a sore leg and a fever. "Oh no," I said to Marc, "I'm getting sick too."

I braced myself for a cold or flu to hit me. I had probably caught some bug in the crowded waiting room. I started vomiting that night. My fever was very high, so I took some Advil, continued to feed Liam, and crawled back into bed.

"How many times can you possibly throw up?" I asked Marc sometime near early morning as the vomiting continued more aggressively. I was very weak and tired, and the ache in my leg was getting worse.

What if it was a superbug? Could it be this strong, this fast? Already I was too weak to take myself to the doctor.

Marc was at work, and Cienna had gone off to school. My parents were helping me take care of Liam, so I called our national healthcare hotline. I ran through my symptoms, mentioning that I felt too weak to get to the doctor.

The nurse on the other end of the line sounded concerned. "You should contact 911 in your area."

After disconnecting my call to her, I immediately dialed 911.

❊ ❊ ❊

My mom and dad were watching Liam in the front room when the EMS team arrived. I told them how weak I was and that I couldn't stop vomiting.

"Well, we can take you to the hospital, but you simply look like an overworked mom," the EMS lady said.

I frowned. What made her think that? Was my house that messy? "But when I called the healthcare hotline they told me I should call 911 and get to the hospital."

"What do they know?" She made a dismissive gesture with her hand.

The male attendant piped up, "If we take you to the hospital, you'll be sitting in the hallways for three or four hours before anyone looks at you."

The female attendant proceeded to tell me that she'd had the flu a few weeks earlier. "With my three kids. I was in the same condition as you, and my husband was travelling. I took some of the new ginger Gravol and it worked. They even have Gravol suppositories. I used it all, and I was fine."

I wasn't convinced. "I have a very strange, strong ache in my right leg."

She tilted her head. "Did you have sciatica in your pregnancy?"

I nodded.

"That's probably it then," she said.

My mom came into the room after they had gone. She had a list of medications from the paramedics that she was going to go get with my father.

Caring for Liam required more time and much more energy than I could muster. Marc was still at work. I was so sick and so tired, all I wanted to do was sleep.

I texted my friend, Bev, and told her what was going on.

She responded right away. *I have never heard you this sick before. I'm making arrangements to come tomorrow morning to help you take care of the baby this weekend, so you can focus on getting better.*

Relief washed over me. I could see my elderly parents were getting tired. Marc had to work, and I wasn't sure how much longer I could take care of Liam. I had no one else to call. Most of my friends had their own children, and some were even pregnant. I wouldn't want any of them to catch this.

I smiled as I tugged the covers over myself, thinking of Bev and how she had driven four hours to see me as soon as she heard we had brought Cienna home. I couldn't help but remember her sitting in my living room, holding my baby girl in her arms. Now she would meet Liam.

I looked down at the little baby lying beside me in the bed. He was so sweet. How many times during the night had I cried with him? I had to get better so I could take care of him. I grabbed for the bowl as the vomiting started again.

After I finished, I called my mother. It seemed like so long ago that they had left.

"Mom?" My head was swirling. "Where are you?"

"We're just paying."

I imagined her standing at the pharmacy counter. "Please, Mom, hurry! I feel like I'm dying here."

❊ ❊ ❊

"Why won't the vomiting stop?" I struggled to get out of bed and walk into the bathroom where Marc was getting ready for work. The pain in my leg was much worse. As I looked at our reflections in the large mirror, the room began to spin around me. For the first time in my life, I felt as though I was going to faint.

"I'll take you to the hospital." Marc reached out and grabbed my hand to lead me back to the bedroom.

There was a strange pounding in my head. It seemed as though I could feel all of the blood coursing through my body.

"I don't think I could make it to the car." I thought of the long walk through the hallways with Liam.

He tucked me back in bed, then picked up the phone and called an ambulance.

❄ ❄ ❄

It wasn't long before a different EMS team arrived. Neither of them attempted to talk me out of going; they just loaded me onto the stretcher.

"I'll wait here until Bev arrives to watch Liam." Marc gently squeezed my hand. "Your parents will follow you to the hospital."

The cold winter air blasted me awake as they loaded me into the ambulance. I could see the front door of our house from the back window as we pulled away and travelled along the streets that led out of our town.

"I've never been in an ambulance in my life," I said to the attendant as she wrapped the blood pressure cuff around my arm. I couldn't believe how bumpy the ride was.

"These things are so temperamental." She sounded mildly frustrated with the cuff. "I just can't seem to get a reading."

I could tell by looking out the window how close we were to the hospital, and I counted the streetlights, willing us to get there faster.

❄ ❄ ❄

Why are there so many doctors around me? I looked around the emergency room they had rushed me into. I counted as many as five medical professionals hovering around me, and I hadn't had to wait for a room.

"Can I have something for the pain?" I pleaded.

Why aren't they getting me something for the pain?

"Get her pants off; she has a rash!" The voice sounded panicked.

"We can cut them off."

Who said that? I looked around.

"I can take them off myself." I pushed my feet into the stretcher so I could lift my backside and pull off my grey pyjama bottoms.

"When can I have something for the pain?" I asked.

A nurse was injecting something into my IV.

"Is that morphine?" The pain was now unbearable.

"No, sweetie, I can't give you anything for the pain; your blood pressure is too low."

* * *

A doctor was standing over me, and Marc was beside him.

I don't remember Marc arriving.

"I'm just going to take a little swab from her leg," the doctor said. "We can use it as a sample to test for infection."

Is he talking to Marc or to me? Why did it seem like I was standing behind him as he said it? I tried to look over his shoulder, but I couldn't see anything.

I wonder when they'll let me go home. My children will be missing me.

8

> "Come to me, all you who are weary and burdened, and I will give you rest."
>
> —Matthew 11:28

MARC'S STORY

"MR. WILKENS, I DO NOT THINK YOU UNDERSTAND THE SEVERITY OF the situation." The echo of the nurse's words clouded my mind until I had trouble sleeping.

I rolled over and stared at the ceiling. Tomorrow the doctors would bring Cyndi out of her coma. It had been over five weeks since she was admitted. *How can I tell her everything we've been through? Will she understand? How can I put it into words that will comfort her?*

The morning Cyndi went to the hospital, I had to wait for our friend, Bev, to arrive to look after Liam, delaying my arrival at the hospital. Cienna was at her friend's house. I didn't feel rushed to get to the hospital, since we were under the impression Cyndi simply had a bad flu. When Bev arrived, I showed her where everything was, handed her Liam, and headed out the door. I was driving down a country road toward the hospital when my cell phone rang. It was the hospital. When I answered, I was quick to mention that I was only ten minutes away.

But that voice. It echoed in my head just as clearly now.

The urgency in the nurse's voice triggered a thought: *This is not just the flu. This is serious.*

Unsure how I'd arrived at the hospital, I found myself with a doctor signing off on paperwork to allow them to medically induce Cyndi into a coma.

The doctor explained that they suspected a bacterial infection was ravaging Cyndi's body, but since the test results would take a few days, they had put her on broad-spectrum antibiotics.

Cyndi's pleading eyes still haunted me. "Please, honey, I'm so thirsty. Why won't they give me a drink?" She reached for my hand. "I don't understand why they won't give me something for the pain in my right leg."

I squeezed Cyndi's fingers to reassure her that they would take care of her. As I let go of her and left the room, the doctors and nurses prepared to place her into a coma and take her to ICU.

The main doctor pulled me aside once again. "Mr. Wilkens, your wife is in septic shock." He explained that her kidneys and liver were shutting down. "She is not going to make it through the night." He lowered his head and stared at her chart. "I suggest you call your friends and family and tell them to get down here if they'd like a chance to say goodbye."

Sitting in the ICU waiting room on a snowy Friday night in February, I was surprised that there was no one else there. The emptiness of the room seemed foreboding. Would I have to raise our children all by myself? I had never felt so scared about the future.

I sat there waiting for our friends and family to arrive. Memories attacked me, reminding me of the life we were supposed to have.

Remembering the joy in Cyndi's eyes when she first held Cienna and then Liam, I broke down sobbing. I thought we would raise our children together. *What will I tell Cienna about all of this?* Liam was far too young. He wouldn't even remember his mother.

She won't die. I shook myself back to the moment at hand. My eyes were drawn to the table beside me. There on the table sat a single book—the Bible.

I touched the chain that carried the cross Cyndi had given me when we first met. I placed my fingers around the cross, sliding it from side to side.

My heart hurt and my head was pounding, I felt as though our lives were spiraling out of control. I had just filled out a form to have my wife put into a coma. They said she wasn't going to make it. How could any of this be happening?

One of the forms had asked if we had a religion; I filled in Christianity. After all, I had been married in a church and was even baptized with Cienna when she was just a baby. I reached over and picked up the Bible. *I call myself a Christian, yet I've never read this book of Christianity.* I'd heard that it was a good idea to read the last chapter of a book to find out how it all ends, so I turned to the last book of the Bible, the book of Revelation, and began reading it.

Slowly, friends and family gathered around Cyndi's bedside to say goodbye. When they arrived, they found her nearly unrecognizable. The medications had already started to bloat her body. She was hooked up to a respiratory machine that was responsible for keeping her alive. An overwhelming sense of lifelessness permeated the room. The blipping lights and sounds of the machine were the constant backdrop to all the hopes and prayers that would be said at her bedside.

My heart broke as I entered the room. She was wrapped up in blankets as if to keep her warm, even though she seemed quite feverish. Her face had bloated and was turning bright red. Her eyes had been covered with cotton balls to prevent the light from penetrating them.

Somehow Cyndi survived that first night. I stayed with friends and family at the hospital as long as I could before returning home, prompted by the nurses to get some rest.

Over the next few weeks, our house would become a revolving door of friends and family coming together in disbelief and support. Tonight, the world buzzed around me. I stood silently in our bedroom for a long time. I looked around at this room I shared with Cyndi. The memories of our time together seemed to be lovingly attached to every piece of furniture. The headboard I had crafted from the wooden door of our first home. A restored antique dresser from Cyndi's grandfather. The photos of us with the children. My heart ached as I broke down sobbing. *Will she leave us here alone?* As if to dismiss the thought, I looked down at our bed where our baby boy, just three months old, lay sleeping. My heart cried out in prayer.

Dear God, I know I have not been a good person or a semblance of a Christian. I have been a sinful man. But Lord, please do not take Cyndi. Our family needs her.

My phone was sitting on the bedside table and I reached over to pick it up. I didn't own a Bible, so I had downloaded one while at the hospital. I stretched out on the bed and listened to the Word of God being read to me as I fell asleep.

✻ ✻ ✻

"Mama!"

I woke to the sound of Cienna's voice. I rushed into the room, and her eyes were filled with tears. I stretched out beside my beautiful little girl and gently stroked her curly brown hair away from her damp face. "Daddy's here," I said soothingly.

"I want Mama!" she said. The tears came harder and were accompanied by pain-filled sobs that broke my heart. She was only five years old. How could I possibly help her to understand? All I could do was stroke her hair and whisper that Mommy would be okay. I believed in my heart that she would be.

"We have to pray for Mommy," I whispered. "She is very sick, and we'll need God to help her get better." I turned away so that she would not see my tears. Eventually, she fell back to sleep.

✻ ✻ ✻

"We have been able to identify the bacterial infection attacking Cyndi," the attending physician said. It was Sunday afternoon, forty-eight hours after Cyndi had been taken to the hospital. She was still fighting to stay alive. Friends and family had taken turns spending nights holding her hand, praying, and speaking to her.

The doctor proceeded to share with everyone that Cyndi had contracted necrotizing fasciitis—otherwise known as flesh-eating disease. He reinforced that they did not expect her to live.

Everyone who had been in contact with her over the last ten days would need to be given a prescription for antibiotics to prevent infection.

I searched my weary brain, compiling a list of those who had been in contact with her, holding her hand or visiting, and immediately thought of our children.

My chest tightened as panic gripped me. It would be difficult enough to raise the children without Cyndi, but I couldn't lose them too. The physician arranged for a local walk-in clinic to test Cienna and Liam immediately.

Dear God, please don't take my children. Please do not let them have this too.

❄ ❄ ❄

I contacted Cyndi's friend, Deanna, who was looking after the kids, and asked her to get them into the car immediately and meet me at the clinic across from the hospital. Twenty minutes later, we walked inside and up to the receptionist. There was a full waiting room, but I was not going to waste any time. I was far too tired and terrified.

"You were contacted by the hospital. My wife is dying." I repositioned my son in my arms. "We're here to have my children tested, and we are not waiting in the lobby."

They took us right in. After a short while, the doctor came in to examine the children.

Cienna had a small pimple on her nose, which caught the physician's attention. She quickly swabbed the children and proceeded to pop the pimple for another sample. Afterwards, Deanna took the kids while I picked up the prescribed antibiotics at the local drug store. I raced back home and administered the first doses to the children.

A day later, I received the call confirming that Cienna had tested positive. Thank God we had gotten the medicine into our daughter in time. I couldn't lose her too.

After a few days, Cyndi was taken into surgery and they removed the necrotized flesh from her right leg, which had started to turn black. She would be left with sixty percent of the muscle and flesh that had previously been there.

I walked into the ICU hospital room and took note of the colour of her hands, turning from light blue to purple to black. Her heart rate was still quite high, and the number of wires and tubes she was hooked up to remained the same.

Sometimes I didn't want to go home, but I needed to be away from the hospital, from everyone. I would drive around country roads listening to my favourite songs, crying to myself and praying. Occasionally I would sit with the chaplain at the hospital and pray. Friends travelled from great distances to help watch the children while I went back and forth to the hospital. After two or three calls in the middle of the night requesting everyone come to the hospital to say goodbye, things had settled down to a very strange sense of routine.

One afternoon when I was picking up Cienna from daycare, her teacher walked over and asked, "How are *you* doing?" My chest heaved and I broke down crying. No one had asked me how I was.

Margaret placed her arm on my shoulder and led me into her office. She took a seat and motioned for me to sit down as I apologized and wiped the tears from my eyes. I told her about Cyndi's current condition and blurted, "I've been reading the Bible and praying."

She smiled softly, "Well, you need to come to church then."

That weekend I walked into church with my children and was greeted warmly. When the prayer list came up on the screen, Cyndi's name was on it. Everyone was praying for her.

❋ ❋ ❋

For ten days, Cyndi's heart had raced at 150 beats per minute. The doctor explained that it was as if she had been running a marathon for a whole week straight. They could not get her blood pressure to rise. I had to sign papers allowing them to inject Cyndi with experimental medication to get her blood pressure up. The nurses told me one shot cost $25,000. They had tried it three times with little success. It all came down to one moment— the moment God revealed Himself to me, showing me He was in control. One evening, after I had arrived home late from the hospital, one of my closest friends suggested that perhaps it was time to think about pulling the plug. He reiterated the medical advisers' prognosis that Cyndi could have brain damage.

"What kind of life will she have? Do you think she would want to live like that? She's had kidney, liver, heart, and respiratory failure. Her limbs don't look good either. It might be time to start thinking about ending her suffering and pulling the plug."

The words slammed into me. It never occurred to me that perhaps her life should be ended. He was only trying to help, and I appreciated his concern, but it upset me.

I got into my car and drove back to the hospital. When I entered her room in the ICU, I was greeted by two nurses. They were accustomed to seeing me and didn't turn me away, even though it was well past visiting hours. My eyes were filled with tears and both nurses reached out and hugged me. Far from being a private moment, I felt that everyone in the hospital had noticed me walking in. My heart raced as I told them, "I need to pray with my wife." I knelt down at her bedside.

Although the room still felt lifeless, I could feel her presence and something else. I reached out and held her now-black and shrivelled hand. Perhaps everyone was right. *What if she doesn't want to live like this?*

Please God, tell me what to do! I don't know what Cyndi wants. It is not my decision to make—to pull the plug and take her life. I have to know if she needs more time, if she wants to live. Father, I can't do this on my own.

I walked blindly downstairs to the hospital chapel and said another prayer there.

The next day I was having lunch at the hospital when I saw my mother-in-law's name come up on my phone. I didn't answer it. How could I tell her the thoughts that were in my heart and head? From the day Cyndi's parents had learned that she was expected to die, they had been very quiet, almost in a state of mourning. Cyndi's father was quite ill with a bad cold and had difficulty getting out of bed. Cyndi's mother visited the hospital often and refused to believe that her daughter wouldn't survive.

After lunch, I listened to the voicemail.

"Marc, I've been busy around the house and I have been told to share something with you." Her voice spoke through my confusion.

She had woken that morning to write in her treasured prayer book. Every family prayer was in it—when Cyndi was hoping to get married and have children, when her son was anticipating getting married. This morning, Barb wrote her prayer down once again: "Please Lord, let Cyndi get well. Bring her home to her children."

As my mother-in-law was doing the dishes later in the morning, she stopped abruptly. Shaking her head, she swore she could hear angels singing. When she was tidying her bedroom, it happened again; it was as if they were singing and speaking to her. She heard some voices and turned to the doorway to see if anyone was there. But she was alone.

"Marc ... you're going to think I'm crazy."

I waited through a long silence until she spoke again. "I've been hearing voices. It sounds like angels singing. I've been hearing it all morning with what sounds like Cyndi's voice saying, 'Please, I want to live. I need more time. Don't pull the plug.'" After hearing this, I stood in the hospital lobby, my shoulders relaxing a little.

God is answering my prayer from last night.

Cyndi's mother had no way of knowing about my night filled with prayer and tears and torment. She was unaware that pulling the plug was even being discussed with friends.

God had revealed Himself and had answered my prayer. I knew now that Cyndi would not die. A great weight was lifted.

I walked back up to Cyndi's room with a lighter step. The burden had been removed from me. She was in God's hands.

The main doctor stood at the nurses' station waiting for me. The same doctor who had repeatedly said that Cyndi wasn't going to make it. Before the doctor could utter a word, I said, "She's going to be okay. You'll see!" We agreed to make one more attempt with the experimental medication to raise her blood pressure.

This time the medication worked.

❋ ❋ ❋

As time passed, I continued reading and listening to my Bible. God was real and He answered my prayer. At night, I would write messages updating our friends and family.

Hello everyone. Cyndi is still in critical condition. She is fighting hard. The doctors are amazed by her. Over the past fifteen hours we have seen her health stop declining and there have been some positive yet very small changes in her condition. They say we must take this hour by hour at this point. We have hope and I know thousands are praying for her. I have received messages from people all over the world who heard about Cyndi and are praying for her. I know some have expressed concern for me and the children. I am trying to be strong for Cyndi and the kids. The kids are doing just fine. We have family and friends helping. I know many want to help us in some way. I will not be too proud to ask for it if needed. Please keep praying for Cyndi. Your prayers have already brought the miracle of her being alive today.

❄ ❄ ❄

I was groggy when I answered a call sometime around midnight. Cyndi had been transferred to a trauma hospital downtown. Her surgeon introduced himself. I steadied myself for the diagnosis.

"Mr. Wilkens, we need to amputate your wife's hands and feet."

"All four limbs?" Paralysis gripped me. "Surely you can save just one limb? One hand…" I pleaded with the doctor, thinking of my wife facing the rest of her life with no hands or feet. What would she be able to do?

"I'm afraid we can't." As the doctor explained the surgery details, I could only think of our daughter. How was I going to tell her?

Days later I sat at Cienna's bedside and gave her the news. She sat there staring blankly ahead, processing the information as best a five year old could.

"But Daddy, won't her hands grow back?"

"I wish they would, honey, but it doesn't work that way. We need to pray for Mommy."

❄ ❄ ❄

Cyndi had been in a coma for over five weeks. Today she would be awake when I visited, and I would have to tell her that her feet, ankles, and most of her calves had been removed. Her hands and wrists had also been amputated. The medical professionals had told me that she was fortunate to have kept her elbows and knees, which would allow her to be more functional.

The doctors also shared that it was likely that Cyndi would be very angry when she woke and heard the news. They warned me to be prepared for the reality that she might even hate me. They suggested I ask her a series of questions to identify any potential brain damage.

My stomach churned as I walked down the long hallway in the hospital. *Please, God, help me to say the right things. Help us to get our lives back.*

Part Two

"Between stimulus and response, there is a space. In
that space is our power to choose our response. In our
response lies our growth and our freedom."

—Viktor E. Frankl

MY SPACE IN BETWEEN

I WAS CRYING. TEARS FLOWED HEAVILY DOWN MY CHEEKS. MY HEART
longed to hold my children.

Someone sat at my head, wiping the tears from my eyes. I could feel the mo-
tion of her hands against my cheek. She had coppery-orange hair and piercing
blue eyes that reflected love.

I heard my words, "I want to go home." Had I said them or just thought
them?

"I know you do." She kindly pulled the hair back from my face. My aching
heart settled as her touch soothed it.

"Why, why?" I searched through the haze.

Her answer was soft. "Sometimes we don't know why these things happen
to us ..."

9

"The Lord is my shepherd; I shall not want."
—Psalm 23:1, KJV

I WISH I HAD KNOWN. I WISH THAT, AS THE AMBULANCE HAD PULLED away from the front doors of my home, I could have looked back and said, "I won't return the same."

The words Marc had spoken echoed in my head. "They had to amputate your hands and feet." I had hoped it was a bad dream, but when I awoke, I was alone. The hospital was dark and dimly lit from the glow of the machines that surrounded me. I could hear them buzzing and whirring as they monitored my life. I couldn't move. I took a mental inventory of the number of wires and tubes connected to my now-small body. Without my glasses, I could only make out the blurry outlines of patients lying in their beds around me. I was in the ICU of a trauma hospital in downtown Toronto.

How could I possibly be missing my hands and feet? I couldn't look down to see them, but I strained to sense if they were there. It felt as though they were. I couldn't make any sense of it.

I searched the darkness of the hospital and was suffocated by a heavy feeling of hopelessness. I tried to hold in the tears that wanted to flow for fear that the nurses and other patients would see me falling apart.

Suddenly, I was back in my bedroom, a young girl of nine years. I was lying on my bed with ballerinas happily dancing across the pink and blue wallpaper around me. In my hand, I clutched a white, leather-bound Bible given to me by my Nana. It had red letters for all the words Jesus had spoken, and I found myself drawn to them, to Him. A bookmark, decorated with lilacs so vivid I could almost inhale their fragrance, marked Psalm 23. I felt compelled to commit it to memory. Every night I would say one more sentence until I had memorized it through and through.

I had used that psalm to carry me through all the pain I had experienced in life or any time I was scared. The words rolled on my tongue, and something deep inside told me one day I would need them.

"Even though I walk through the valley of the shadow of death ..."

I stopped. Why couldn't I find the rest of it? I knew the words that came next would surely bring me comfort. My head was imprisoned in a thick fog that apparently prevented me from capturing more than one sentence.

My frustration grew into anger. *Why would you do this to me, God? To me? What did I do to deserve this? Haven't I always been good? Haven't I been through enough? Really? Haven't I? I have always had faith in you! Why me?* I wanted so badly to turn my head and scream into my pillow; instead, I screamed in my head over and over again—a long, anguished, gut-wrenching scream. I should be at home in my bed, nursing my son. But I was here, alone and isolated. How I wished this ache in my heart would go away.

Oh please, God, I cried, *let this be a dream. Take me back. Transfer me to my bed, and when I awake, let my children be there in my arms.*

Perhaps, given my muddled thoughts, I believed that, since it seemed like just yesterday that I was holding them, I could embrace yesterday and bring it back to me. If I closed my eyes and went back to sleep, maybe, just maybe, I would wake up and be at home, holding my son with one hand while gently brushing the hair from my daughter's face with the other. Floating around in this space, it seemed as though I was sinking into a slimy pit. It was so easy to close my eyes and float into the darkness.

When my eyes opened, I was greeted once again by photos of my happy family looking back at me, hanging from the IV pole. The photos represented a sense of normal that had been replaced by the void in my heart. They had been taken in December, only three short months before. In them, my arms were wrapped lovingly around my son and daughter. Would I ever be able to do that again?

When someone experiences loss in a way that rips apart her life, her heart begins to feel like a war zone that is being repeatedly bombed. The wounds heal, but the next loss reopens the wound even wider.

My heart was a minefield. It had been blasted by loss of fertility, loss of hope of what my marriage would be, infidelity, and the loss of trust that accompanies it, and now … Our marriage was already strained. How could we possibly get through this? How could Marc look at me with love? How could he find me attractive? How would anyone find me attractive? I could spend the rest of my life alone. What kind of life would I have?

I thought back to the white light I had seen. It was so clear to me that it was God. I had no doubt that He was coming for me. Or was I going to Him? How could I describe to anyone what I had seen? I so wanted to tell Marc or my mom.

A nurse with brown eyes and hair braided in cornrows interrupted my thoughts. She stood above me and explained that she had been taking care of me.

I tried to speak, but there were no words.

She reached up and removed an empty bag of medication hanging from the IV pole. "We're waiting for a plug to come from downstairs." I shook my head, trying to communicate that I didn't understand. "You've been in a coma and had a tracheotomy. We require a specialized plug to help you to speak. It hasn't arrived yet, but we're hoping it comes up soon." She hung a new bag of clear fluid on the pole.

I stared at the ceiling. I had no voice? I couldn't ask where Marc was, or how he was coping, let alone where my children were and how they were doing? I was trapped, a prisoner in my own head.

She turned to me. "Your family is here to see you. Would you like them to come in?"

Actually no, I didn't. I wanted my mother. I didn't want anyone else to see me like this. Maybe, if they didn't see me, none of this would be real. I mined deep into my heart, looking for strength. Finally, I found the courage to nod.

It appeared as though the people approaching me walked through a foggy haze as they entered my room. My mom came in first. Her small frame contained a heart into which had been poured the most faith I have ever encountered. The welcome sight of her short, salt-and-pepper hair and warm brown eyes made me want to reach out and console her. As she stood beside my bed, I ached to touch her. I longed for someone, anyone, to hold my hand. To grasp it and console me as my mom had done when I was a little girl.

Dad is just under six feet, and as he entered, his hazel eyes reflected his joy at seeing me alive. I prepared myself for him to make a silly joke as he always did to comfort me. But he didn't. Bev followed my parents, oozing positive energy and leaving no room for anyone to question her joy and relief that I had not died as the doctors had predicted.

My little room quickly filled with people. I scanned the small space. My parents and Bev, my nurse and the social worker assigned to me, all stood around me, yet I felt completely isolated. How could they possibly understand what I was feeling? I was alone. I had no hope of speaking to them. I couldn't tell them all of the things that were on my mind. My words were trapped inside my head, screaming to get out.

With compassion and a desire to help me try to communicate with my family, the nurse and social worker brought in a large whiteboard with letters on it and asked me to spell out what I was trying to say by simply pointing out the letters. I raised my bandaged arm and, not looking at it, pointed to the M.

Bev knew immediately that I was asking about Marc.

"He's doing well." She rested a hand on my shoulder. "It's really important that you focus on you right now. Don't worry about everyone else."

But I was worried. I worried that there was no way my Marc could possibly handle this. It wasn't how he was made.

The darkness was calling. By simply turning my head and closing my eyes, I found a way to communicate. People would walk away and go home, and I didn't have to pretend that everything was okay.

❋ ❋ ❋

A few hours later, my nurse received a new plug. The one that had arrived earlier hadn't fit, but this one did. The first sounds I made were gravelly as I tried to ask for "w-water." I was so thirsty, as if I had been walking in a desert for months.

"We can only give you ice chips to start," said the nurse.

"My husband?" I asked.

She nodded. "Would you like me to call him and let him know that you are able to speak?"

"Yes, please." Relief flowed through me. I could speak.

She came back a short while later to let me know that Marc was on his way.

I let the effects of the medications take me away.

❋ ❋ ❋

Marc was standing over me when I woke. His eyes were bright with intensity. "Hi, honey," he said. The sound of his loving voice caused the pain in my heart to rise up again.

"Do you know where you are?"

I looked around and managed to respond, "Hospital."

He smiled that soft smile. "How old are you?"

My forehead wrinkled. "Forty-two." I was starting to get confused and frustrated. *Why is he asking me these questions?*

"Do you know where you live?"

That seemed like a strange question. Of course I knew where I lived. I answered him begrudgingly.

He leaned in closer, his eyes reflecting that look of intensity once again. "I have to ask you these questions to make sure you're okay, honey. The kidney dialysis and everything that your body has been through could have caused brain damage. But clearly you are going to be all right." He hugged me as he started to tear up. "I'm so glad you're back. We have two children to raise together."

He pulled out his cell phone and started showing me photos of the kids. Cienna smiled back at me, posing in a pair of my boots. Liam's baby face grinned at me, and a small tooth peeked through his gums. How many moments was I missing? The wounds in my heart reopening, I turned away.

I had so many questions. I had so much to ask him and tell him about. I needed to hear that he was going to stay with me like this. The intensity of the love in his eyes was unfamiliar to me. Every time he spoke words to me it was as if he was attempting to convey the depth of that love to me. His eyes reached into my soul, saying, "I love you."

I raised my bandaged arms. "But look at me ..." My voice broke.

Marc didn't hesitate; he just gazed at me with loving intent. "Honey, I fell in love with your soul, your heart, and your eyes, not your hands and feet."

The words I had longed to hear touched my soul deeply. When he left, once again I allowed myself to float back into that darkness, even as I wished he had carried me away with him.

10

"Never will I leave you; never will I forsake you."
—Hebrews 13:5b

WHEN I WOKE AGAIN, THEY HAD MOVED TO ME TO A SMALL, MAKESHIFT room. Instead of walls, there were curtains, and I could hear my neighbours coughing, conversing with their visitors, and crying for help. It was morning, and the hospital was bustling with activity. Nurses hurried to check on their patients before breakfast arrived and rounds started.

The weight of the hospital air seemed different here. When mixed with the cries of suffering patients, it carried a heaviness of despair and hopelessness. It seemed thick and dense, making it difficult to breathe in.

When I looked down at the floor, I could tell by the shadows created by light streaming through blinds that there was a window behind me. Was it sunny outside? How long had it been since I'd seen the sun? As the nurses and hospital staff bustled around me, I realized that, for the first time in my life, I had no sense of time. I didn't know what day it was, where my children were, who was with them or holding them.

Marc had told me that he'd hired a nanny. The knowledge that someone else was holding the baby boy I had prayed so hard for seemed unfair and heartbreaking. Panic overcame me. *Where is my daughter?* A longing overcame me to reach out and grab my child to my chest and hold her. But I couldn't. I would have to get this feeling of panic under control. I fought back the tears and took very deep breaths.

I tried to recall the look of love in Marc's eyes and that feeling of hope I had gone to sleep with. But what if he was just saying what he felt he should say, words he believed I wanted to hear?

My mind struggled to process the fact that I had been in a coma for five weeks. For me, no time had passed. It was as though I had gone to sleep one night and woken up the next. It seemed like just yesterday I had held my baby boy, my hands gently massaging his head in that intimate way that mothers do. My heart ached at the thought of my son and my little girl. How would I take care of them now?

Would I ever be able to hold my son in my arms again? How much pain had my daughter endured while I was not there to soothe her? How would I take care of my children? Would I ever brush my daughter's hair, feed my son, push them on a swing? How would I even take care of myself? My mind was assaulted with thoughts of all the things I had done as a mother that I couldn't do now. Once again, I found myself in that familiar position of hitting rock-bottom. It was as though I was tumbling down a black tunnel, the darkness covering me and smothering me as I fell. I tried to reach out with my hands to grab the sides of the tunnel, but I couldn't. I couldn't even find the energy to take my next breath.

I lay there, unable to move, as people walked by, avoiding eye contact with the woman who had no hands or feet, only tubes sticking out of every part of her body. My family was far away, I couldn't hold my children in my arms, and my heart was lying on the floor, shattered. I had no idea how I would ever put it back together again.

I was paralyzed by atrophy, and my body was far too weak to move, so I went back to sleep. In sleep I did not have to face that ache that started in my stomach and reached up into my heart. The open wounds in the mine-field of my heart.

❋ ❋ ❋

"We have to move you again." The nurse called for an orderly. They had been moving me on a regular basis, slightly to one side with a pillow propped up under my back, and then slightly to my other side. Each time they moved me the pain was excruciating, as though every nerve ending in my body was raw. I had learned to hold my breath and pray, *Please, God, give me the strength to get through this.*

I was missing a chunk of my right leg where the necrotizing fasciitis had entered. There was no skin there. Eventually I would need to have that skin replaced. In those moments of movement, the pain in my raw, open, wounded leg matched the pain in my heart, leaving me breathless.

As I braced myself to be moved again, the nurse said, "Your parents are here to see you." My heart fluttered. My parents were there. Familiarity. I couldn't wait to see my mom again. She always made things clear for me. She would know the answer to my question.

I contemplated her as she entered. I had always thought I would take care of her as she aged. That was likely no longer possible. Who would take care of my sweet little mom? I was holding so much inside, not wanting to worry her by revealing the pain in my heart. I put on a brave face, but I was bursting with questions.

She looked at me, her soft smile reflecting the love mothers carry. Once again, I tried to will her to reach out and hold my hand, or where my hand used to be. Suddenly I couldn't keep it in any longer. The burning in my heart gushed right up and out of my mouth before I had a chance to think about it.

"Mom, why would God do this to me?" There they were—the words I longed to say.

Her eyes widened. "You don't think God did this to you, do you? God would not do this to you."

I wanted to believe her. But why hadn't he stopped it? How could he let such a horrible thing happen to me? How could he take my children from me? I had worked so hard to build this family. My heart and soul were with those two children. Wave of overwhelming pain crashed over me again. The waves were difficult to fight.

"Mom … please, hold my hand." She tentatively reached out and lovingly rubbed what was left of my arm.

Once she left, I thought back to what she had said. "God will make it right." She had taught me all my life that God that could do anything. But how could He make this right? My hands and feet would not grow back. *Was it even possible to make this right?* If He didn't cause what had happened to me, surely He would fix it.

11

> "'For I know the plans I have for you,' declares the Lord, 'plans to prosper you and not to harm you, plans to give you hope and a future.'"
>
> —Jeremiah 29:11

I FELT AS THOUGH I HAD BEEN WAITING FOR THIS DAY ALL MY LIFE. "I'm bringing the kids down to see you this weekend." My heart started to beat as Marc told me his plans. I wanted to hold them in my arms, to pull my daughter's head to my chest and stroke her hair. I ached to tell her that it would all be okay.

Marc looked around the room. "I don't think I should bring them into the ICU. Maybe your nurses have some ideas about where we could meet."

The nurses suggested a small waiting room outside the ward.

The last week had been a week like no other in my life—a week of floating in and out of darkness, questioning God, and searching for some type of understanding.

I had met my physiotherapist, my social worker, my surgeons, and more nurses than I could remember. Because I could not lift my head to look around, I learned to measure my days and nights by the amount of light in the hospital ward and by the shift changes of my nurses. Just as I would start to feel comfortable with one nurse, the shift would change and I'd have another one. Very seldom did I have the same nurse two days in a row. That made the loneliness and isolation feel even greater.

My social worker arranged for me to be able to call home every night. The nurse would dial the phone number for me, then set the phone on the pillow beside my ear so I could talk to Cienna and hear all about her day. At first she stood there, holding the phone to my ear, but I felt terrible having long conversations and monopolizing her time, so I learned to hold the phone between my shoulder and ear. I would grow weary fast, but hearing my daughter's voice was my motivation. I wanted so badly to be there for her.

I had fought so hard this week.

My current nurse had blue eyes and long brown hair. Today was the second day she had attended to me, and I had grown very accustomed to her. She was full of warmth and kindness. For what seemed like hours, she had tried to brush a five-inch knot out of the back of my very long hair. She looked at me, her blue eyes reflecting the warmth in her heart, and softly said, "I have to cut your hair."

Not my hair too? I took a deep breath. That deep-down strength was there, I just had to find it. I dug into my heart.

"Cut it." I tried to hold in my tears.

"Are you sure?"

"Yes."

She had to *saw* through it more than cut it. I felt each stroke and every single chunk that fell from my head. Finally, she came out from behind me and held up a blood-encrusted, blonde-streaked knot. My long hair was gone.

My hair had always made me feel so feminine. Why did it have to be taken from me too? What had I done to deserve this?

"God didn't do this to you." Mom's voice echoed in my head.

I turned my head and let the tears flow. I didn't want anyone to see. I cried for the hands that would no longer grow long fingernails. I cried for the manicures I would never share with my little girl. I cried for the toes that would never feel grass beneath them again.

❋ ❋ ❋

When I awoke in the dimly-lit hospital, I peered down to the table at the foot of my bed and saw a face I had been dreading. I had watched her. The way she looked at me every time she passed by. A look I did not have words to describe, yet. She was one of the nurses.

I tried to smile.

"I'm going to give you a wash tonight," she said as she proceeded to run water behind me and fill up a pan. In my little four-by-eight cubicle, I hadn't encountered anyone who looked at me strangely up until this point. From the outside world, I had only seen Marc, my parents, and my friend, Bev. My resolve to stay strong was rapidly weakening.

She set the basin of water on my tray table and removed my hospital gown. Her hands matched her demeanour—rough and impatient.

I looked down and for the first time I could see scars all over my body. Wires came out of everywhere. There was a large black wire in my groin, along with several new scars, which I had no memory of receiving. More wires were connected to my chest and hooked up to a machine that monitored my heart rate. The blood pressure cuff on my arm inflated once an hour to take a reading. I knew I was on a catheter and kidney dialysis, but I had no idea how those were connected up. Worse yet, a tube removed all of my solid waste. That knowledge reminded me that I had been stripped not just of my physical parts, but also of what was left of my dignity.

I blinked back tears. Another tube went into my nose and down to my stomach so I could receive nourishment.

As the nurse washed me, I focused on the feeling of the water, trying to visualize it washing away some of my sadness.

She washed down my chest and around all of the wires connected to it. When she started washing my private female parts, I turned my face away. Would I ever be able to wash myself?

God, is this how the elderly feel? All their dignity snatched away? The ache returned to my heart. This time it was not just for my lost dignity, but for all my loved ones who would suffer the same way as they aged. Would they lose their voices as well? I thought of my parents. I couldn't stand the idea of anyone having to go through incredible loss like this.

I begged for sleep to help me escape.

❊ ❊ ❊

The nurse wasn't done with me. In the middle of the night she walked back into my room and turned on the light above my bed. "Your bandages need to be changed tonight." She studied the bandages on my arms where my hands had been.

I had been able to get some sleep, so I summoned a smile, ready to make an attempt to melt her demeanour.

She was slowly unwrapping the bandage on my right arm when I heard it. A sound at the back of her throat as she shook her head from side to side, a tsk. She continued to the bare arm, exposing my stitches. Each layer seemed to bring a shake of her head from side to side and that sound. She kept peering down at me with a look I couldn't quite identify. I searched for a memory that might tell me what it said, but I'd never seen that look in anyone's eyes before. Then it dawned on me. In a way that crushed every ounce of resilience and ounce of strength I had, I realized it was pity. She was contemplating me with a deep, resounding expression of pity.

To emphasize the point, she continued to shake her head as if to say, "Your life is over."

I wanted to scream, to shake her and yell, "My life is not over. You do not know me. God will fix this. You will see!"

My heart felt a sudden rush of strength. God would show her.

Please, God, let me get my life back. I can't do this alone.

※ ※ ※

Today I would see my children again. They were on their way. I tried to still my heart, afraid it would leap from my wounded chest. The hours seemed to slowly tick by. I tried not to dream about what our first visit would be like for fear I would be disappointed. I was determined I would attempt to hold Liam, although I had no idea how. I couldn't wait to kiss my girl's face.

The nurses helped me get ready. I had spent time sitting up in a wheelchair, preparing my body so that it would be strong enough to sit while the children were visiting.

I was still connected to an oxygen tank by a tube that ran into my neck. Every time I was moved, the tube had to be disconnected and reconnected. The nurses wrapped a scarf around the tube so it was well hidden from the children. They settled me in the chair and wrapped blankets around me. I was grateful for their efforts to restore my dignity and smiled at them as I slid my arms under the folds of blankets. In spite of all our preparations,

I was nervous and scared as they rolled me out of the unit and down the hallway. Would the children know me?

"Hi, Mama," Cienna said as I was pushed into the room. Without hesitation, she came over and kissed me on the cheek. It was the most precious kiss.

"Hi, honey!" Marc leaned over to kiss me with Liam in his arms. I wanted so badly to hold my baby boy, but focused my attention on my daughter. It seemed like just yesterday I had seen her, but as I scrutinized her, I realized she wasn't the same little girl. She had grown.

"Look, Mommy, I lost another tooth." She proudly displayed a smile that showcased her missing front tooth. A pang shot through me. I had always been there for every event in her life. I pushed away the thought, refusing to allow my thoughts to travel that road.

Marc sat down on the couch at the opposite side of the room. Cienna crawled around on it and continued to chat the way five-year olds do. She told me about school, her best friend, and life. I was so thankful that she did not seem bothered by my hidden missing limbs. I took a moment to study my husband. He had a diaper bag slung over his shoulder as he held our son on his lap. He bore no resemblance to the man I once knew. He had become "Mr. Mom." Mom was my job—the job I had waited to do for so long—and now I couldn't do it. All of this seemed so unfamiliar and unfair. Would I ever feel normal again? I looked at Liam. He had grown so much that he was not the baby I had held in my arms. He had changed.

What other moments would I not be there for? Would I miss him eating his first foods, taking his first steps? The doctors were saying that I would be here for a year. *There's no way I can be here that long.* I needed to find a way to get home to my family. I strengthened my resolve and finally got the nerve up to ask, "Will you bring Liam to me?"

Juggling Liam in his arms in front of him, Marc walked over to me.

I held my breath in anticipation. I wanted to kiss my son's cheek, rub his head. As my husband moved closer, holding Liam just above me, time seemed to move slower than usual. My heart was full of anticipation.

Did I think he would know me right away? Don't they say that babies know the smell of their mamas? He recoiled from me and cried, his arms clinging to Marc's neck. He did not want to be with me. His mother.

Before long, I sensed that the children and Marc were growing restless. The discomfort of sitting upright for so long had moved from dull to immobilizing. Although I wasn't ready to let them go, my body needed rest. Cienna and Marc said their goodbyes and the nurses rolled me back down the hallway to the place that had become my temporary home.

Although I had no way of knowing why God was putting me through this, my heart would not give up. I had worked too long and hard to get these children. I had fought to come back; I had begged to come back. God had allowed me to live. As they transferred me to the bed, I was overwhelmed with sadness. Words echoed through my head as I screamed at the top of my lungs, deep inside, *I will not give up.*

12

> "You keep track of all my sorrows. You have collected all my tears in your bottle. You have recorded each one in your book."
>
> —Psalm 56:8

IN JESUS' TIME, ROMAN WOMEN COLLECTED THEIR TEARS OF PAIN AND suffering in small jars. Faced with the loss of a loved one, women would weep into small clay pots. The amount of liquid in the jars represented how much the women loved the one who had died. When the jar was placed into the tomb, the tears would slowly evaporate.

King David tells us that the Lord records our tears. He knows how many we have cried. Perhaps, like a loving father, He reaches His hand out and catches them for us.

When I look back upon my life, I realize that I would need a library to hold all of the tears of joy and sorrow I have cried. I would spend much of my time wandering in my library, brushing my fingers gently over each of the jars sitting on the shelves and reflecting on the moments described on their spine-like labels.

The larger jars would have bold labels with my children's names. They would hold the tears I cried while longing to have them, and finally holding them.

As I slowly walked through my library, I know I would often find myself at the largest shimmering gold jar. After picking it up, I would walk to my favourite chair. Of course, the chair would be sitting beside a window overlooking a garden. There I would rest, cradling the tears from that inconceivable day when my life was forever changed.

I would not want to have any of the liquids evaporate. Especially not this one. I would never want to forget the knowledge that washed over me in that hospital. In spite of the overwhelming pain and confusion, I knew I was not alone. I clung to that truth and to the knowledge that there can be beauty in pain, and His name is Jesus.

※ ※ ※

My parents came often, and my dad would help me with the prescribed exercises to strengthen my muscles. One day, as they were leaving, my physiotherapist walked in. "How do you feel about trying to sit up at the side of the bed today?"

My nurse was unhooking my IV tube, leaving the needle in my arm. I nodded. "Sure." I was both eager and scared. This would be the first step toward getting home. How hard could it be?

She reached over and released a valve at the bottom of my bed. Slowly my mattress started to get smaller. As the cushioning air released from my mattress, I felt myself sinking closer to the bottom of the hard metal bed frame. My confidence wavered.

Was my life deflating too? My hopes and dreams dissipating and floating away from my grasp?

"Can you turn on to your side?" The physiotherapist interrupted my musings.

I pushed the assailing thoughts away and attempted to turn over. I failed. The flat, hard surface I was now lying on prevented me from moving.

"No, I don't know how." I looked up, puzzled.

Standing at the foot of my bed, she must have sensed my confusion and inflated the mattress one third of the way back up. As my body rose up with the air, my confidence rose too.

"Now try." She had a calm and reassuring voice. I instinctively reached out my hands to brace myself on the bed, but … "How?" I pleaded, holding in the tears.

"You may have to use your elbows." She moved behind me and placed her hands on my back.

She gently pushed as I dug my left elbow into the bed and tried to roll over. I floundered as I attempted to dig my foot into the bed. Her gentle push was enough to roll me over. I had done very little, but was on my left side.

Even slightly inflated, the bed was hard on my hip.

Without thinking, I again reached out my hands to pull myself up and once again faltered.

I had no hands or feet. Each movement relied on them, and they were gone. How would I ever do anything? I wanted to be able to figure it out, but I was frozen. I didn't know how to do this on my own. *Please, God, help me.* I had never felt such desperation.

"Maybe you can pull yourself up." My physiotherapist lifted the rail on the side of the bed and locked it into place.

I reached my arm out and stopped. *How?* Then it came to me. I wrapped my right arm around the top of the bed rail and pulled.

"That's it." The physiotherapist moved behind me once again, bracing my back and easing me up.

"Are you dizzy?" She came around the bed to stand in front of me. "Do you think you could get your stumps over the edge?"

I contemplated the question. I would have to maneuver my left leg out from under me and pull myself up with my arms. I shifted my left arm to the rail, swung my left leg out, and pulled. I didn't have enough strength.

"Keep breathing."

When did I take my last breath?

I gritted my teeth and pulled harder, slowly rising.

"There ... you did it." We both exhaled.

I sat in my spot triumphantly, although my stumps dangling where my feet would have been threw me off balance.

"I'm dizzy."

Her hands eased me back down onto the bed.

What was ahead of me? I could barely sit on the side of the bed, and I wanted to walk again. The crest of the mountain I was climbing seemed unreachable.

The bed was inflating, my body rising with it, limb by limb.

Please, God, be my strength.

❋ ❋ ❋

The double doors opened and I was pushed through, exiting the ICU trauma unit. The nurses had spent all morning getting me ready for my visit with the children. They had once again put me in a wheelchair with four-inch padding. My legs were covered with blankets, but this time I felt comfortable enough to leave my arms in my lap, exposed.

I had been speaking to Cienna on the phone every night. "We are coming back to visit you this weekend, Mommy." My days were bombarded with nurses checking vitals, medicines, and feeds through a tube connected to my stomach. I had been plagued with vomiting and uncontrollable hot flashes and felt incredibly weak. But when I heard my daughter's voice on the phone, I was reminded of what I was fighting for.

The hallway appeared much longer than I remembered. Before long, we were turning into the small waiting room.

Marc held Liam on one side of the room, and Cienna stood on the couch directly in front of me. As soon as she saw me come through the doorway, she jumped off the couch and ran toward me.

I opened my arms for her to hug and kiss me. Her eyes left my face and proceeded down my arms. She stopped.

Her beautiful brown eyes widened and she retreated to the couch on the other side of the room.

Marc came over and kissed me on the cheek. He was speaking, but I couldn't hear his words. My eyes would not leave Cienna as she remained on the far side of the room. I wanted to walk over and console her, but … I started to cry.

Marc tried to console me by making small talk. He attempted to encourage our little girl to come over to me, but she wouldn't.

My own child is afraid of me.

Marc quickly realized that there was no point in carrying out the sham of a visit. Liam did not want to be anywhere near me either.

As they rolled me back down the hallway, away from my family and back into isolation, I sobbed uncontrollably. I had held my tears in for so long. I had put on a strong front, ensuring that the nurses around me would not know the depth of the pain I was in. But when the tears came, it was as though they had been building up for years. I spent hours crying and fighting the sense of hopelessness that was invading my soul. I had lost so much.

God, how could you do this to me? I couldn't turn onto my stomach, grab my pillow, and cry into it; I was essentially a shackled prisoner in this position and this bed. I settled for turning my head to bury my face into the pillow beside me.

I was overwhelmed by what I was facing. I would have to re-bond with my children and re-learn how to do everything from brushing my teeth to walking. The pain gushed from the pit of my stomach to the crater where my heart was as I silently cried, *My son doesn't even know who I am.*

An answer came ... a small, still voice from deep inside: *You know what to do. You've adopted; you read all about attachment parenting.*

I paused, reflecting on the many books I had read in preparation for adopting, especially the chapters on attachment parenting.

How long would it take? I imagined myself walking around on prosthetic legs with the baby strapped to my chest. Was that even possible?

"But how will I know ..." my chest heaved as I searched for the right words, wiping the tears away with my arm, "... when he bonds to me?"

Another answer came: *You'll know when he cries for you.* Memories flashed before my eyes of the look on Cienna's face when I dropped her off at preschool. In spite of struggling against the thought that I was abandoning her, I was always reminded, when I saw that look, of her love and of the gift I had been given in being her mom.

Images of Cienna growing up and getting married flashed before me. I would be there to see it. That was a gift too.

While I was still wiping away my tears, the nurse came in. "It's my dinner break now; I can read to you, if you like." She held a book in her hand.

When I nodded, she sat down in the chair beside my bed, shifting to find a comfortable position before opening the book.

"*For you created my inmost being; you knit me together in my mother's womb. I praise you because I am fearfully and wonderfully made.*"

I stared up at the ceiling, rolling the words around in my mind. *I was fearfully and wonderfully made.*

The nurse read on, but the words continued to echo in my head. Would God have created me for this? I was overwhelmed with the revelation that great intention had gone into creating me. As I listened to the words, reinforcing the truth that I had been created with purpose, it was as though a finger reached across and placed the first bandage on my heart.

My wonderful nurse looked up at me from the book and smiled. Her eyes were warm and her fingers were laced in the pages as she continued with a poem by Russell Kelfer:

No, that trauma you faced was not easy,
And God wept that it hurt you so,
But it was allowed to shape your heart,
So that into His likeness you'd grow.[1]

She lifted her head and we made eye contact, both smiling.

She jumped up from the chair. "I'm going to photocopy that for you."

As she ran off, I tried to process what she had read. I was created with intent. God had a unique purpose for me. I studied my tiny, broken body, hiding under a hospital blanket, minus the bumps at the bottom of the bed where my feet would have been.

When the nurse returned with the poem, she taped it onto the inside rail of my bed. I simply had to turn my head to see the words. "No, that trauma you faced was not easy, and God wept that it hurt you so."

God wept for me. My tears started flowing again.

God wept. How I wanted to shout it through the hospital, waking everyone with that incredible news. I was not alone.

Over the past few weeks, many nurses had prayed with me, reminding me that I was not alone. What had I thought they meant? Now I knew.

God, is it possible that your heart is broken too? Please help me put my heart back together again.

I imagined Jesus standing beside my bed, picking up the shattered pieces of my heart and lovingly placing them into the spot where the crater had been hollowed out.

---

1   Russell Kelfer, "You Are Who You Are for a Reason," http://185218.web14.el-exioamp.com/life-lessons/read/selected-poems-by-russell-(readprint)/you-are-who-you-are-for-a-reason (accessed August 28, 2017).

Oh God, I've been so lonely here, and for most of my life. The words brought a sense of relief. Had I been holding them in?

I had gone from being a little child, moving from place to place and struggling to make friends, to a betrayed woman lonely in her marriage.

Please God ... don't make me do this alone.

A voice responded, *You are never alone.*

Warmth erupted, His love filling my soul, flushing out my anger and hurt.

He who had suffered most, comforted me.

I had almost died at the age of forty-two. All the things I had thought were important—things I had been chasing for the last few years—were now irrelevant or pointless. None of them could have taken away the look of pain in my daughter's eyes.

I hadn't been expected to live. That was clear to me. Friends and family had told me how sick I had been. Every single breath I would take from this point on would be yet another gift.

I don't have the strength for this fight. But God does.

I read the words on the inside of my bedrail and was encouraged once again. Now I knew. He would carry me through, holding my hand. And maybe, one day, I would shine again.

13

"I knew your face when you entered the room.
I knew your arms when they embraced me and called me 'beloved.'
I felt your hands wipe away my lonely tears as you spoke,
'My child, I mourn with you, I cry with you, your tears are precious to me.'"

—Cyndi Desjardins Wilkens

THE BIBLE TELLS THE STORY OF A WOMAN WHO REACHED OUT IN FAITH 2,000 years ago.

I often imagine this nameless woman, lying in her bed the night before her life was about to change. Was she excited, or nervous? Truly, she had nothing more to lose. She was isolated from her family. She had spent every last coin on physicians, trying for a cure. Nothing had worked. The twelve years of bleeding had drained her body, her savings, and her dignity.

At that time in history, women with medical issues were separated from their family and labelled *unclean*. No one, not even her children or her husband, would be allowed to touch her.

As she rolled over in her bed, attempting to calm the anxiousness and fall into a restful sleep, did she wonder what this Jesus of Nazareth would be like? Had she heard about the many miraculous things He was doing? He had performed miracles of healing such as no one had ever seen.

The next morning, as Jesus made his way through the throngs, she slowly crept toward Him, pushing her way through the crowd. Her heart must have been beating out of her chest, the sound of it muting the loud, enthused voices of the people around her. With a shaking hand, she reached out and touched His clothes.

She knew immediately the constant flow of blood had stopped. She was instantly healed.

Jesus wasn't angry when he discovered who had touched His robe. Instead, He said, "Daughter, your faith has healed you."

How many nights had she spent tossing and turning and grieving the loss of her life? More than she could have counted, probably. And countless more stretched out ahead of her. Until that moment she reached out and touched Him.

❋ ❋ ❋

I spent a month in the ICU of St. Michael's Hospital. My "space in between" lasted almost two weeks. I didn't stop grieving the loss of my life, but suddenly I was grieving with a faith that, even though I could not imagine how, God would redeem it for me.

Many times I experienced foreshadowing of the rest of my life, the looks of pity or sadness I would be given, and the strength it would require to focus on the things that I was able to accomplish, instead of all I had lost.

Today I was celebrating my forty-third birthday. I tried hard not to think about where I should have been spending my birthday—at home, surrounded by my children and family. Would I have had a party? Just four short months ago, I had arranged a surprise fortieth birthday party for Marc.

My parents visited first, bringing birthday cards, love, and news from home. I was happy to see them. "Marc will be here after work," my dad shared.

I was still being fed by a tube, but before my parents arrived, I had been X-rayed to determine if I could handle solid food. Since I'd had a tracheotomy, the doctors needed to ensure that I could safely and effectively swallow again. The results confirmed that I could. The nurses purchased an ice cream cake, and my friends, Maria and Cindy, as well as Marc, soon joined me in my room.

"How are you?" Cindy moved closer to the side of my bed.

I forced a smile. "Good." Inside the truth lingered; I didn't tell her about the excruciating pain I underwent daily as I was moved around in my bed, when I sat up in a chair longer in order to condition my body, and as I did my prescribed exercises to strengthen my arms.

I also didn't tell her that twice a week, healthcare workers changed the dressing on my right leg. The first time they came in to replace the bandages, I felt as though every nerve in my body was being cut away. The doctors chose to anaesthetize me for the many dressing changes that followed. I was secretly terrified of every procedure and every surgery. I had almost died; each procedure could result in the same, couldn't it?

Marc pulled up two chairs for the girls and stood behind them. I shifted slightly to the right, attempting to get more comfortable. I looked at my husband. "Can I have an ice cube?"

Marc reached over and slid one into my mouth. I seemed to be parched all the time. I let the liquid float around my mouth for a while, hoping it would satiate my thirst.

I wanted to share with them what had happened at rounds that week, but how could I articulate it without sounding ungrateful? In the secret place in my heart, I was terrified. I was fearful that I wasn't courageous enough to get through every moment, that my family wasn't strong enough to support me. I had worked my way up in business without showing fear, believing it was a sign of weakness. If I told them how scared, tired, and full of pain I was, would they think my faith in God was slipping away? Would they worry that I couldn't handle this? It would be easier for them if I let them think I was doing great, that I didn't experience daily pain and humiliation as strangers bathed me and moved me around and discussed my case between them while sharing very little with me. Should I share all of that, or just try to carry it myself?

As part of my morning routine, I watched the doctors congregate at the foot of my bed. One morning, as I was trying to focus on their conversation, I was drawn to a movement behind them. Was it her? The coppery-haired woman who had stroked my head while I was in the coma? My heart filled when I realized that it was. She walked behind the doctors. I smiled, hoping she would see me. She stopped and gazed at me intently with her bright blue eyes. "We were very worried about you, but now we know that you are going to be okay." She smiled a warm smile once again and walked away, disappearing as quickly as she had appeared.

The corners of my lips turned up as I thought of her. I hoped to see her again.

Marc set the cup of ice cubes back on my tray table and resumed his position behind the girls. "Cyndi is scheduled to have skin grafting surgery next week."

My stomach flipped at the thought. They would remove a thin layer of skin from my left leg and place it on my right, where both skin and muscle had been removed due to the necrotizing fasciitis. In addition to the pain, I was concerned about my heart. The doctors and nurses had mentioned that my heart had failed in the coma. They had put me through numerous tests to confirm that it had not been damaged. What if I was too fragile to undergo another operation? How does a heart come back from failure? *Please, God, let it be strong.*

An older man walking around the unit and playing guitar drew me back to the present. The nurses sent him over to sing "Happy Birthday" to me. A hospital room may not have been where I thought I would spend my birthday, but so many had worked hard to make sure it was a good one. Although my heart was still very sad, I fell asleep that night reflecting on the laughter and love of friends.

❋ ❋ ❋

My next two weeks at St. Mike's Catholic hospital were a whirlwind of milestones. Whether I was ready for surgery or not, one week after my birthday, I was rolled into the operating room.

Sensing my fear, one of my nurses walked over and reached out to hold the end of my arm. "Would you like me to pray with you?" I nodded gratefully as I thought back to the day she had first approached me. I had been embarrassed at the thought of others seeing me pray. Now, I couldn't wait for that hint of peace to surround me before my operation.

After the surgery, one of the first friends to come in and visit was a young, female co-worker.

"Would you like me to cover the tubes leading into your body?" the nurse asked me.

I thought about it for a while. I was humiliated by the number of tubes running in and out of every crevice in my body; however, as vulnerable as it made me, this was and is my reality. If anyone who visited could not endure the sight of me, I needed to know now.

As soon as my colleague walked into the room, I knew I would likely never see her again. Her expression and body language made it clear that she could no longer stand to be around me, and I held back tears during the short, awkward visit.

I responded to the isolation, loneliness, and heartbrokenness that set in afterwards with a strength I didn't know I had. And I made a decision: I refused to allow anyone but God to tell me what my life would be.

✹ ✹ ✹

"I have some good news." My nephrologist came in and sat down beside my bed. He visited almost daily to discuss the kidney dialysis I was on.

He folded his hands and leaned in. "Your creatinine levels are back to normal." He smiled, but I was perplexed, until he explained that creatinine in my blood was a way to measure how my kidneys were performing. "We will be taking you off dialysis." His smile widened.

I could barely breathe. We had thought I might be on dialysis for the rest of my life. "What's today's date?" I searched my memory, counting the days since my birthday.

He paused before rising from the chair. "The twenty-third." He disappeared into the ward.

March 23. *Oh thank you, God. I will forever remember this day!* I couldn't wait to tell Marc.

I sank back on my pillows, my heart filled with joy and gratitude. I had made it through surgery, and my heart and kidneys were strong. I could feel the presence of God all around me. *Thank you, God, for letting me live.*

14

I WAS TRANSFERRED BACK TO SOUTHLAKE HOSPITAL FROM ST. Michael's by ambulance at dusk. The doctors had simply walked in and said I was too healthy to stay where I was. The idea of changing hospitals terrified me. I knew that I would have to get accustomed to a completely new routine, and new nurses and doctors.

By the time they rolled me through the foyer of Southlake, memories were flooding my mind. This was the hospital where I had given birth to Liam and the place I brought my children when they were sick. I had spent a month here myself in a coma, fighting for life.

The hospital was in night mode with the lights dimmed. A deafening silence welcomed me.

Through the quiet, my heart seemed to speak. *This is the place your questions will be answered.*

I wasn't concerned about questions as to how prosthetics work and why all of this had happened. I had come to the realization that I may never know why. No, deeper, more difficult questions plagued me. The kind of questions that start deep in the heart and surface with a resounding boom. The ones that drive a person to search for answers as a whale might search for the surface to breathe in air.

I couldn't help but think of my children. They would be sleeping right now. Here, they were a short fifteen-minute drive away. How would Cienna respond to me the next time she saw me? A deep desperation for her to accept me resided in my heart. The desperation for my son to recognize me travelled just as deep into the recesses of my heart.

And what of Marc? We had not been alone yet. He had said he loved me, but there were always nurses in the background, other patients around. How was he really doing? It was baffling to think of my husband handling this situation. How could the man I knew withstand what we were going through and what we would have to face? Did he really want to be with me?

I took a deep breath.

They rolled me into a room that was set up to closely monitor patients after surgery. Three curtained sections opened onto a central desk area where two nurses were stationed. The sounds of the other patients, combined with the various monitoring machines, were a vast contrast to the silence that had first greeted me.

I could sense the nurses' discomfort as they greeted me. Had they ever cared for someone with no hands and feet?

I rolled my head to the side, thinking about the young man who had been my attendant in the ambulance. I had tried to make idle conversation with him. The look of surprise when he first saw me made his discomfort with me painfully evident. I wanted to scream, "Please treat me kindly. Please treat me as you would have if I was ..." the tears started, "... whole."

Would I be treated differently for the rest my life?

Please, God, tell me I won't face this reaction from everyone I meet.

I gazed up at the ceiling of this new room. I was becoming accustomed to staring up at ceilings. Before all this happened, how would I have responded to someone like me? Would I have been kind? *You would probably have averted your eyes and walked away,* my heart responded. Shame washed over me. *No! I would have been kind.* Tears were starting again. Surely, I would have been kind?

The nurses had not yet come to see me. There was a patient next to me who required attention and didn't speak English. I tried to think of something I could say to make the staff feel more comfortable around me.

I sighed heavily, the type of sigh that was an attempt to expel all worries. *Just breathe.*

As a prisoner in bed for over a month, I learned how to pass the time. If I was frustrated that I couldn't get up, I would fight it by setting goals, writing storybooks in my head for the children, and praying.

For every fear that entered my mind, I would take a deep breath and find an answer. How would I get Cienna to be comfortable with my arms? Perhaps if I could use them as puppets? I imagined painting faces on them. I could call them Ren and Stumpy. I chuckled to myself, imagining what it would be like introducing them to my kids.

My thoughts were interrupted by my first visitor in my new "home," a tall man with blue eyes and blond hair who walked in and stood at the foot of my bed.

"Cynthia?" He came over to sit in the chair beside me. "My name is Derek. I'm a pastor and a friend of Marc's."

My forehead wrinkled. I searched my brain, but we had no friends who were pastors. He sat down on the chair beside the bed, his warm eyes on me. "What did you do to that man to give him such faith?"

Now I was very confused. Maybe he had the wrong Cynthia. Who was he talking about? I was the one who had faith in our marriage. I was sure this situation would be too much for Marc. It was just a matter of time.

Derek folded his hands in his lap. "The nurses downstairs—the ones from ICU—have heard that you've returned, and they're excited to see you."

"That would be nice. I'd like to thank them." Marc had told me how committed the nurses were to my care.

I chatted with the pastor for a few minutes before he excused himself. Slowly, over the course of the evening, I was introduced to many members of my care team. Eventually my bed was surrounded by ICU nurses, the same ones who had taken care of me when I was in a coma, fighting for my life. I tried to remember them, looking into their eyes and searching for a memory that I could not find.

Eventually sleep crept in as I thought back to what the pastor had said to me. *What did you do to give him such faith?* Was he talking about my Marc? Was it possible that Marc was doing better than I thought? I took another deep breath and rustled the bottoms of my legs into the sheets.

Surely God was helping Marc through all this. I hadn't done anything. It could only be God.

Something about those deep breaths and the hospital night mode brought me peace, reminding me once again that God would make everything right.

15

"The Lord will guide you always; he will satisfy your needs in a sun-scorched land and will strengthen your frame. You will be like a well-watered garden."

—Isaiah 58:11

DOES A FLOWER HAVE A SURVIVAL INSTINCT? AS IT STRIVES TO REACH for the sun and slowly opens up, does it have to struggle to live? When the rain drives down upon it, does it have to fight to stand? Every time I steadied myself, ready to move through a new challenge, more rain would pelt down.

My first days were filled with meeting my care team of physiotherapists, occupational therapists, even social workers, as well as my relocation to a private room.

I was questioned by psychiatrists, psychologists, and social workers, all trying to determine if I was a risk for depression. I probably saw a dozen people concerned with my mental health.

As the hospital social worker entered my room yet again, I braced myself. As she questioned me, I told her what I could about my life experiences.

How many medical professionals had I given my life story to? How many more would I have to?

"Have you had any suicidal thoughts?" There it was. *Maybe I'm depressed and I don't know it.* I searched my heart and found only faith and determination that I would get home to my children, my life.

"No, but should I experience any, I will let you know right away."

My nurse entered. "We are going to get you up for physiotherapy."

How would they transfer me from the bed to the chair? At St. Michael's Hospital, orderlies had lifted me from one to the other. The nurse called for assistance, and soon another nurse came into the room. They had me roll to one side and then to the other as they maneuvered a large piece of fabric underneath me.

"This is called a Hoyer lift; we will get you into the sling and connect you to that lift above the bed." The first nurse pointed to a hydraulic machine attached to the ceiling.

Once I was securely in the piece of fabric, they lowered the hook and connected me to the machine. Slowly I was lifted up and out of my bed, across the room, and into the wheelchair.

As the lift carried me across the room, frustration built up in me like a geyser ready to explode. *This should not be happening.* A deep breath later I was praying, *Please, Lord, let this be temporary.*

They rolled me through the ward and down to the gym. I placed a gentle smile on my face, a smile that I hoped conveyed: I am kind, I am approachable, but I am not to be pitied.

Once I was in the gym, my chair was placed in front of a large padded table. My physiotherapist stood beside me. "Try moving each hip separately to transfer onto the bench."

I shifted each hip forward while resting my arms on the wheelchair and in a short time I was sitting on the bench. *I'm getting stronger.* That was the most I had moved since entering the hospital.

The gym was occupied by several patients. My physiotherapist helped me to lean back. "Let's start with some exercises to strengthen your legs." She grabbed a pillow and positioned it under my neck. I lifted each leg up for several repetitions. A lady was exercising her arms from a wheelchair beside me. I returned her smile. *This is so futile. How can leg lifts enable me to walk again?*

Across the room another physiotherapist was working with a young man. He was learning to walk again, but each step was strenuous and after four or five he collapsed into a chair, exhausted. What had happened to him? I focused on my leg lifts while pondering his situation. His legs didn't work. I would get legs to enable me to walk. *I need to have faith.* I pushed on. *This will have an exceptional end result, the incredible joy of walking again,* I reminded myself with each rise and fall of my leg.

Later, as the nurse fed my dinner to me by spoon, my stomach started to churn. Tonight I would see the kids. *How will they react to me this time?* I tried to brace my heart.

I took inventory of how my daughter would see me. Although the tracheotomy tube—along with most of the rest of the tubes that had been inserted into my body—had been removed, and a gauze bandage covered my neck, I was still being fed through a tube in my nose that led into my stomach.

My hospital room was decorated with cards and flowers. It was almost cheery.

The sound of their voices travelled down the hall. How I longed to run and wrap my arms around my children. My heart beat a little quicker as they drew closer.

Cienna bounded in first with a smile on her face. "Hi, Mama!"

Behind Cienna, Marc walked in with the Filipino woman he had hired to be our nanny, the one who was with my son every day. Although I had readied myself to meet her, nothing could have prepared me for the wall of pain that washed over me when I saw this stranger with the long, dark hair carrying the little boy I longed to hold.

"Come." I scooted over, patting the empty space on the bed. I had planned ahead. Cienna's favourite TV station was on.

"Lie down beside me and let me rub your back." I smiled lovingly. Cienna cautiously stretched out beside me, careful not to touch me at all.

Please, God, hear my prayer, I pleaded as I gently rubbed her back. Warmth flowed through the end of my arm as my skin made contact with the soft pink shirt that covered her back. My heart was beating so fast I was sure everyone could hear it. "See honey? Remember how I always rubbed your back before bed? It's just like before." Gradually her little body relaxed. I wanted to weep for joy and the knowledge that I would never forget this answered prayer. As I held my breath and waited patiently, I imagined myself wrapping my arms around her and holding her close.

Although there were a lot of conversations going on around me, I was only aware of two things—my daughter, who was slowly moving closer to me, and my son. Although he was just across the room, he felt miles away.

After quite a bit of time had passed, when Cienna was comfortable, I asked the nanny to let me see my son.

Marc picked him up, sat him up on the foot of the bed, and put a toy down beside him so that he would have something to play with.

A wave of familiarity attacked me. The wave had built up slowly when Cienna first entered the room. I was overwhelmed with the desire to run over and wrap my arms around her, the way I had always greeted her. But things had changed. Looking down at Liam, I realized he was wearing clothes I had picked out for him. I had gone shopping for outfits just after Christmas. As his mother, I had lovingly picked them out, thinking about the times I would have him wear them. Now I couldn't even dress him. I pushed back the assault.

I had also bought him the teething ring sitting beside him. It had many rings that made a rattling sound when it was shaken. *How can I pick it up with no hands?* Liam's eyes, big and blue, focused on the ring as I reached my right limb out and touched the cool plastic surface. His hands shook in anticipation. Encouraged, I grabbed it between my stumps, shaking it until I heard that familiar sound. His eyes twinkled as he grinned. My heart leapt with hope.

Time stood still while he was occupied. But then he started to fuss, and panic rose in me as he held out his arms for the nanny. The sinking of my heart must have been evident on my face, because Marc moved in quickly and lifted Liam off the bed himself.

"He's probably hungry. Let's get him a bottle." He wasn't really hungry; he showed little interest in the bottle. Inside, I pleaded for Marc to give him to me. *Surely I can comfort him. I am his mother.*

I glanced down. Cienna moved a little bit closer to me.

"Do you see Mommy's arms?" I swallowed back the lump in my throat. I would not cry in front of my children.

She nodded.

"This is Ren." I held up my right arm. "And this is Stumpy." I waved my left arm around. "If you touch him, he's very snuggly." My left arm had a lot more flesh than my right arm.

My daughter placed her fingers lightly upon my arm. It took some time, but she eventually grew comfortable enough to watch TV while holding on to my left arm. I smiled. *Stumpy will grow to be her favourite, I just know it.*

My son was not settling, and I could sense Marc's agitation. "Okay, Cienna." He strapped Liam into his stroller. "It's time to get home and ready for bed."

The words cut right to my heart, but I pushed back the pain. *They can't stay forever.*

Marc kissed me quickly, but he appeared preoccupied.

As soon as they left the room, I let the tears flow. How long would it take for my son to know me? How long? Oh, how I resented the woman holding him. Hopelessness threatened to set in. I had become familiar with that attack, and I fought it, smiling at the memory of Cienna holding my stump.

Is that how it will feel to hold hands now? I imagined walking along the sidewalk with Marc grasping my stump.

Experiences in life such as holding hands, and the warmth that creeps up the arm in response, are so powerful, so intimate. Once again, I found myself reflecting on the sensation of my toes in the grass and the little blades sticking up between them. Would I forget those feelings? Was it necessary to forget them so that I could move on? Would the memory of them always bring this longing into my heart? Tears streamed down my face.

In an attempt to distract myself, I turned my attention back to the TV.

Visiting hours would soon be over, and the hospital was preparing to go into night mode, when the lights would be softer. The door of my room creaked open. I stiffened, hoping the nurse wouldn't notice I had been crying.

But it was Marc. As he walked toward me, I looked into his blue eyes and started to cry again. This was the first moment we had been alone together.

His eyes were also flowing with tears as he motioned for me to make room and then stretched out beside me.

The room was silent. We had no words; we only stared at each other for a long time, and then he rested his hand on my cheek.

"This is so hard …" he whispered, and we continued weeping and gazing into each other's eyes.

This was the attack of the unfamiliar, the constant burning, yearning for what life had been, pondering the unknowns and uncertainties.

"I put the kids to bed and came back as soon as I could." His voice was thick with exhaustion.

I took a deep breath. This was my chance to say all the things that were in my heart, and yet, where would I find the strength?

"Honey, if this is too much for you, I understand if you don't think you want to be with me anymore." There I had said it. It was done.

He pulled his head back and looked at me quizzically before smiling softly. "Honey, I love you. I told you before that I didn't fall in love with you for your hands and feet." The look in his eyes was intense. "I fell in love with your beautiful soul. What kind of man would I be if I turned and walked away? I love you, honey."

He stayed beside me for a little while longer, both of us trying to comfort the other. Two sojourners attempting to hold onto one another in the midst of this unfathomable journey.

16

"I sought the LORD, and he answered me; he delivered me from all my fears."

—Psalm 34:4

My hair was freshly washed and wet when my parents arrived for a visit. Because I was bedridden, washing my hair was not an easy task. The nurses would bring in special pans. They covered my head in plastic and washed it as I lay there. It took quite a bit of time, but it always made me feel refreshed.

My dad was eager to help and offered to blow dry it for me. Slowly and gently he ran the brush through my hair as he dried it. He was careful not to harm the large sores left on my scalp as a result of being immobile for so long. He hesitated at every brushstroke. Was something wrong?

He held the hairbrush for me to see; the bristles stared back at me, covered in my hair. He lifted his free hand, which was now shaking. His fingers were wrapped around a large chunk of my hair. My eyes scanned along the many strands and found the ends attached to a large, ugly scab.

"I think your hair is falling out," he said softly.

"It's probably just because of the sore on my head."

Sitting at my bedside, Mom nodded her head and smiled comfortingly.

After they left, I settled back on the pillows and thought back to the many mornings I had woken to find long pieces of hair on my pillow and scattered through my bed. There was no denying it. *My hair is falling out.*

Was I being stripped of everything I held pride in? I loved my long hair as a lion loves his mane. I had worn my hair long since I was a child. I would run my fingers through it several times a day. My mind flashed back to the numerous times in my life I had been complimented on it. *Will I go bald too?* I couldn't reach up and feel its texture with my fingers, so I asked the nurse to bring in a mirror.

She brought in a small mirror and set it in on the table. The face that looked back at me was very different than the one I remembered. My brown eyes that were always smiling now carried a sunken appearance. Where did that hollow look come from?

The photo of our family beckoned me from above the bed. It had been transported to the new hospital with me and re-attached to my IV pole. I was much smaller now, and that was reflected in the shape of my face.

Who will I be now, God? I pushed the mirror away; I had seen what I needed to see.

Later that evening, the children visited. Once again, Cienna walked in and climbed up on the bed with me. I'd had the nurse turn the TV on, and her favourite channel waited for her.

Liam was in his stroller on the other side of the room. An idea was brewing.

"Cienna," I spoke softly, "Liam doesn't know who I am." I leaned in closer to her. "Can you tell him I'm Mama?" My eyes travelled across the room and rested on Liam. "Maybe *you* could show him who I am?"

My daughter jumped off the bed and marched across the room. She had easily taken on the role of big sister, particularly in my absence. She picked up her little brother and set him down on the bed beside me.

"Liam, this is Mama." She waved her arm in a dismissive gesture. "She looks different because she cut her hair."

She returned to her favourite TV show as I sat there with one arm wrapped around Liam, chuckling as I looked up at Marc. Our eyes met with amusement. Yes, that was why I looked different. Because I had cut my hair.

17

"Like a snow-cooled drink at harvest time is a trust-worthy messenger to the one who sends him; he refreshes the spirit of his master."

—Proverbs 25:13

I WAS WAITING OUTSIDE CIENNA'S SCHOOL TO PICK HER UP. I COULD SEE her peeking out, but there was a man with her. The man exuded the essence of danger.

Several doors dotted the outside of the building, and the man peered out one of them periodically, but he would not let her come to me.

I was frantic.

He is trying to take her. I reached for her, but no matter how hard I tried, I could not stretch my arms far enough to touch her.

I woke up from my dream sweating. Unable to shake off the helplessness that threatened to overwhelm me, my heart slid back into that slimy pit of distress and despair.

It was a weekday morning, so my daughter would be at school. How long had it been since I stood at the door and waited for her to come home and share the exploits of her day?

Would I ever feel normal again?

I struggled to focus on the things I could do, however short the list. But the darkness of loss was starting to set in again.

Please, God, help me. I am so tired of trying to be strong. Please carry me.

The sadness in my heart that day must have been noticeable, as I was visited by many social workers. Two of them sat at my bedside, kindly listening to the outpouring of my dream. I released the fears of my heart that I had not yet given a voice to.

How can I get closer to my children?

How will this affect my daughter for the rest of her life?

What if she can never forgive me for getting sick?

We were so close, what if I can't get that back?

I directed the attention of the social workers to a picture on the wall that Cienna had drawn of me, reflecting on the day she had brought it in. "I drew this for you, Mommy." She had proudly waved it in front of me.

She placed it on my lap. It was a drawing of me. My hair was long and I was smiling.

I did not have hands, only rectangular, box-shaped arms.

My legs also ended in rectangles with no feet.

At first I was horrified. This was how she saw me. This was me.

But my eyes were drawn to those legs. She had coloured them a sparkling, shimmering gold. I smiled, even as the tears flowed. My daughter saw me in a way I could not yet see myself.

Did she really see me that way? Shimmering gold?

I thought back to the woman I had viewed in the mirror. Although I had come to terms with not understanding why this was happening to me, secretly I could not look at this body of mine and call myself "beautiful."

I certainly did not feel outwardly beautiful. Inside, I was mostly the same. Mostly. But there was a tiny part, down deep, that felt like a small seed struggling to grow. Struggling for more light.

Cienna saw me in a way I couldn't interpret. Did my shimmering legs reflect that light?

I couldn't help but recall her reaction to my request to show Liam who I was.

"She looks different because she cut her hair …" Was it possible that, other than that, I was no different to her?

When they returned the next day, the social workers brought in a desk and chair to place in the corner of my room. Using large letters, they posted up the words, *Cienna's Corner*.

They placed markers and crayons all over. That night when Cienna visited, I couldn't wait to show her the new creative corner. She started drawing and creating immediately.

As I watched her carefully colouring, I thought to myself, *God, tell me she's going to be okay.*

She looked over at me and smiled a big smile as she held up a picture she had drawn of her and me.

My gaze shifted back to the picture of the woman on my wall with shimmering legs.

Please, God, let me shimmer like that again.

My five-year-old little girl had brought the word *beautiful* back to my heart.

❋ ❋ ❋

Days ran into nights. Days filled with exercising, strengthening, and visits from my parents, doctors, and friends and family.

For a change of scenery, my parents often took me to lunch in the hospital cafeteria. I wouldn't eat much. I still had a feeding tube that ran at night, making my stomach feel full all day. Friends and family would bring me food, but as a result of the medications, my taste buds were not functioning.

After my parents finished their lunch, they would roll me out to a lounging area outside of the cafeteria where I would sit and watch people. Visitors often found us there, Mom reading her paper and sharing the highlights with me as Dad nodded off in the comfy lounger. A small sense of normalcy.

"Hey, the nurses told me you'd be here." My brother-in-law, Carl, walked up and hugged us. "I called Marc, and he said you'd be up for a visit." I hadn't seen him since he had come to visit at Christmas. That was four months ago. My stomach churned as I looked for signs that my appearance caused him any distress. I sighed when I saw that he had none. I had learned to search all visitors who hadn't seen me limbless yet. As I studied everyone chatting, I recalled Marc telling me that Carl was one of the family members who had visited me in the coma.

Two strangers approached, a man and woman. The man's gaze made contact with mine.

"Cyndi?" I returned his kindly smile as I nodded. My gaze fell upon the name badge he wore. *Is he also a chaplain here?*

"I'm Pastor Michael and this is my wife, Shelley." He gestured to the lady beside him. She was holding a large pink drink with a big red straw.

"We're friends of Marc's from Lakeside Church." I searched my memory again. *What is the name of the church Marc has been attending?* Was it the same?

He smiled at my parents. My dad stood and shook his hand, then Carl introduced himself.

Mom touched my arm. "The church that Marc's been going to."

I nodded.

Shelley approached me and held out the large pink cup. "We stopped on the way and bought you a strawberry milkshake." I reached out to grab it between my stumps. She stepped back to stand beside her husband. "We thought it probably wasn't something you could get here." I lifted the cup to my lips and took a sip from the straw. The flavour danced on my tongue. *I can taste it!*

"How are you feeling?"

"Good. I'm getting stronger every day."

Everyone was smiling now. Clearly my enjoyment of the milkshake was evident.

"We have some more visiting to do." Their eyes were full of kindness. "You will remain in our prayers." They turned and made their way past the lounge area and disappeared into the lobby.

I turned back to Carl, "How are my nieces and nephew? Give me all the news." As he shared the highlights of their teenage lives, I couldn't stop the thought, *How will they respond to me?*

Much later, after my visitors had left, I lay in bed, thinking about my day. How many pastor friends did Marc have? What had happened to him while I was in the coma? Would I go to his church one day? I smiled as my lids became heavier. *Thank you, God, for my family, for letting me live, and for strawberry milkshakes.*

※ ※ ※

Later that week, Cindy and Maria visited and coaxed me into having my first big meal. They hand-fed me a sub sandwich. My taste buds were working again. As I began to eat more meals, the nurses removed the feeding tube. My body was now tube free.

Anticipating the return of my appetite, my team had been working on making me a glove that would allow me to feed myself. Because my amputations were below the elbow on both sides, I was more likely to be able to accomplish simple tasks such as feeding myself with the assistance of a cuff that wrapped around the end of my right residual limb. It fit similar to a blood pressure cuff, and had a pocket to insert a fork or spoon handle.

My occupational therapist slipped the cuff onto my arm and, after several attempts to find perfectly shaped and angled cutlery, she succeeded. She watched as I was able to scoop and lift pasta to my mouth. Sensing my excitement, she asked, "Would you like to be alone?" I eagerly nodded and she left the room.

My wheelchair faced the window in my room. Every day I watched the traffic go by, wishing I could be out there in the world.

I lifted the pasta to my mouth and cried. This was the very first thing I had done for myself. I couldn't walk. I couldn't grasp hold of anything. But I was feeding myself. I no longer had to face the indignity of having to ask others to do it for me. *No, now I can do it myself.*

I finished the plate of pasta faster than I thought possible. Then I looked down at my lap, where most of my meal was now nestled. I laughed. It wasn't a loud laugh. It was a laugh that seemed to resound deep within my spirit. A laugh I shared only with God.

I couldn't wait to tell Marc when I spoke to him on the phone later. "I fed myself."

"That's great!" There was so much excitement in his voice, I couldn't help but smile. "You're doing so well." I could hear his pride. "I bought you an iPad and adapted it for you; I'll bring it tonight and we can try it out together."

He was moving faster than I expected. I had just eaten my first meal. I wasn't ready to start typing out sentences on an iPad. My throat tightened, but Marc had planned it all out. He had searched for a specialized stand that would put the device at my height and angle.

As soon as he arrived, Marc inserted a stylus into the cuff I had used to feed myself, and in no time, I was typing. Clearly inspired by the joy she saw in me, Cienna reached out and drew a big heart on the screen with the words, "I Love You."

"You're still coming to visit for Easter, right Mom?" she asked. I had been requesting a pass from the doctors. A pass would enable me to go home for a few hours.

"Yes, honey, I can't wait." I held her close to my heart. These visits were a balm to my soul. Although it hurt to watch my family walk away from me, after they had gone I was filled with a renewed determination to continue doing everything I could to get well.

❊ ❊ ❊

Two long weeks passed before I was loaded onto the wheelchair van and driven home.

Cienna stood on the doorstep, jumping up and down.

I read her lips through the window of the van. "Mommy's here; she's here!"

Marc appeared at the front door, holding Liam and smiling.

I wanted to run to them. To open the door, step out, and wrap my arms around them. But I waited for the driver to come and roll me out in the wheelchair.

Too many sensations bubbled up inside me to be contained in my heart. Excitement, frustration, and nostalgia threatened to overwhelm me. Emotions swirled to the tips of my missing fingers and toes.

It had been a rushed morning as the hospital staff prepared me for my first visit home.

When they came to change my bandages that week, I smiled and endured it. The donor site on my leg was not healing well. The area where strips of skin had been removed from my left leg for skin grafting on the right would not heal. Aware of the pain, the nurses drowned the bandages in saline water. Regardless, as they were peeled off, they would take the newly-formed skin with them. I would be left with bloody red stripes down my leg and in a raw pain.

Knowing that I would be visiting home helped take my attention off the pain. I tried to visualize being pushed into the front lobby. Would I smell the aroma that was home? I dreamt of turning to Marc and my children and saying, soon, very soon I am coming home for good.

"You're here, Mama!" Cienna's voice called me back to the moment. She rushed over and kissed me on the cheek.

I studied the door of my house. The door I had gone out through three months before.

There was a sudden frenzy of hospital staff and friends who had arranged to be there to assist Marc in getting me inside. I was tipped backwards in my chair, lifted up the stairs, then rolled through the double doors. Once in the foyer, I peeked into our living room as Marc pushed me past it and into the kitchen.

While Marc thanked our helpers, I sat in the room I had loved spending most of my time in. How many dinner parties had I hosted here? How many carefree, joyous hours had we passed in this room? I replayed the happy moments in my head as I waited.

The kitchen was *my* spot in the house. I lovingly and sometimes furiously cooked all the meals. I knew where everything was, since I had placed it there. How many times had we had friends over who would ask, "Can I help you with anything?" I would point to a chair and say, "No, just keep me company." How I loved those times.

I frowned. A sense of betrayal crept in. Things had been moved around. My favourite coffee maker had been replaced. Nothing seemed to be the same. I peered past the kitchen into the open doorway of the dining room. The table was piled high with papers. When had the family last dined together? I scrambled to grasp hold of something familiar. I searched for that scent of home, but couldn't find it. My house even smelled different.

Marc returned with the kids. He pushed me into the living room as Cienna carried her little brother. After he'd situated me in front of the couch, Marc took Liam and set him on a blanket on the floor. The blanket was scattered with his toys, many I had lovingly purchased in anticipation of his arrival, and some that had once been Cienna's. Each toy carried a memory.

How I would love to walk into the kitchen and make a cup of coffee. With mug in hand, I would walk back and pick up my son, holding and loving him. I would snuggle down with him on one side of me on the couch and Cienna on the other. Life would be … normal again.

I blinked. Cienna was telling me about her weekend. "Mommy, today we learned Jesus died on the cross for our sins." Marc was now attending church every week, and my daughter was learning the gospel.

I thought of her words, "for our sins." Our sins. I had never thought of myself as a sinner. I thought Jesus died for murderers and thieves. But as I looked back on my life, I saw so much sin. I had such a desire to please everyone but God. I placed my faith in people. I had wanted so many things … but not Him.

The afternoon with my family flew by. As Cienna showed me her artwork, I kept looking at the clock. The wheelchair van was going to be late picking me up, but would still be arriving far too soon.

I wanted so badly to get on the floor with Liam. I longed to walk up the steps to the washroom and down the hall to my bedroom. I would lie there and refuse to let anyone move me.

When the van pulled up, I realized the kitchen and living room were all I would see of my home this time. Marc lovingly wheeled me through the foyer and back out the doors. I focused on the beautiful time I had spent with my little girl. *I can be strong by simply thinking of her.*

"Give me a hug, honey." I opened my arms. Cienna's gaze was on the driver, who was lowering the ramp to the van.

Marc moved in to hug me. "We'll come and visit you later." He kissed me on the cheek, then stepped back and slid his arm around Cienna. The driver rolled me into the van and secured my chair to the floor.

The door slammed shut.

That was it. My sentence seemed so final. Through the window, I caught a glimpse of Cienna, crying for me now. Was she wondering why I couldn't stay? The thought tore at my chest. I had come to terms with the fact that I might never know why any of this was happening to me, but how could I expect my little girl to grasp that truth? As we pulled away, her small shoulders drooped, and she sobbed for her mama.

Back at the hospital, after I'd been transferred back into my bed, I collapsed in exhaustion. My nurse was kind and gentle, as though she sensed my sadness. I buried the deepest of my emotions until she left.

As soon as she was gone, the reservoir, filled to overflowing, could no longer contain my tears.

The walls that held in my suffering came down. My chest heaved with sobs as I flashed back to the image of my daughter crying on our front lawn. *Why do I have to go through this?* I furiously punched my arms against the mattress.

I had been in this state for eleven weeks; the entire time I had been filled with an aching need to see my children, worry for Cienna, tears over the loss of my son, and so much fear. *I am tired, God.* I lay there, my body, mind, and spirit exhausted.

Words called out to me. Words I had asked to have attached to the side of the bed. I wiped away the tears with my arm so I could see them clearer. *"No, that trauma that you faced was not easy, and God wept that it hurt you so."*

I was not alone. He was crying with me.

I had been thrown a life preserver. I clung to it. With no hands, I wrapped my arms around it so tightly I could not let it go. I continued reciting by memory.

"But it was allowed to shape your heart, so that into his likeness you'd grow."

18

> "I will extol the LORD at all times; his praise will always be on my lips."
>
> —Psalms 34:1

LIGHT FLOODED THROUGH THE LARGE WINDOWS IN MY NEW HOSPITAL room at West Park Rehabilitation Hospital. They overlooked five acres of parkland in the middle of Toronto. The glass was cracked open just enough to hear the birds singing.

A small vase harbouring freshly-picked lilacs rested on the window-sill. One of my nurses had brought them in for me. When God created the lilac blossom, did He envision the scent travelling from person-to-person, bringing the essence of His healing touch? He must have known how many would breathe in that sweet aroma and be reminded of special moments, or even of their own gardens.

The lilacs that grew in my back garden every year were likely now in full bloom. I had been lying in a hospital bed for 14 weeks. I longed to walk barefoot in the back garden, wandering around, enjoying the scent of fresh flowers. I retraced each step of my backyard in my mind so that I would not forget.

My nurse had brown, curly hair and brown eyes. She had taken me on a tour upon my arrival. The park-like setting of the hospital carried a cacophony of bird songs and the scents of flowers and trees mingling together. Rooftop gardens and patios with ample seating had been placed conveniently around the property. Many patients wandered the property by electric wheelchair.

It was difficult to accept that I would soon be in one of those electric wheelchairs. Although I was anxious to have control over my mobility, I was nervous. Truly, I would've liked to have skipped the chair and moved right on to new prosthetic legs so that I could run home immediately.

I had been given a wonderful sendoff at Southlake Hospital, including a surprise party with cake and beautifully-written cards. I promised to walk back in one day on my new legs.

A few days before I left, my physiotherapist strode into the room and stated plainly, "Today we are going to try to do 3-point kneeling."

"Ok," I agreed, not sure *what* I was agreeing to. "What is 3-point kneeling?"

"We are going to get you to stand on your knees." She leaned into me as she pushed me down the hallway.

My heart started to race as I transferred onto the bench. I had been strengthening my muscles with leg lifts and arm pulls, but standing on my knees was intimidating.

She set a chair in front of me. "I want you to move from all fours, place your elbows on the chair, and pull yourself up to stand on your knees."

I took a deep breath. Part of me wanted to just say "no thanks." I struggled onto my elbows and knees. My atrophied muscles were unresponsive as my body had not yet been in this position. With every limb shaking, I shifted my right arm to the seat of the chair.

Terror swept over me. My chest tightened and I struggled to draw in air. How would I get my other arm to the chair without falling flat on my face?

I can't believe I'm doing this.

"Try putting your other stump on the chair and then pulling yourself up." The therapist moved closer to me. I could sense her excitement.

Didn't my face reflect enough of the growing fear in my heart? She wanted me to go further?

Numerous times over the last few months I had been visited by friends who would say, "If anyone can do it, you can." Where did that faith in me come from?

Please, God, help me. Please hold my hand. I am so scared. I can't quit now. With all the strength I could muster, I lifted my arm and plunked it on the chair.

I let out an exceptionally large sigh and lowered my head onto my arms on the chair seat. I had done it. *Thank you, God.*

"Okay!" The therapist broke the silence. "Now let go of the chair and stand as tall as you can on your knees."

What? I can't let go.

Adrenaline was pumping through my body, and every part of me was shaking. All eyes in the gym studied me. If I failed, it could let them all down, but if I succeeded, they too would be lifted up.

With a silent prayer, I straightened up on my knees, as tall as I could, my stumps resting on the chair to provide balance. Very slowly I dropped my right arm down to my side, then my left. I stood there shaking on my knees for what felt like an eternity.

I don't know how long I can hold this. Every muscle in my body vibrated in revolt.

Finally, my therapist said the words I was waiting for, "You can come back down now."

I managed to maintain my balance as I slowly lowered myself back to the chair and rested both arms on it, barely refraining from hugging it.

She smiled. "You are gifted with strong balance."

Before I knew what was happening, I was back on all fours and sitting on the bench. It was over. I felt as though I had just climbed a mountain. I had been terrified, but I prayed, I pushed through, and I did it. A thought kept trying to push into my consciousness, nudging at me. *If it's that hard to stand on my knees, how difficult will it be to walk again?*

❋ ❋ ❋

The most exhilarating and terrifying advantage of being at the rehabilitation hospital was that on the weekends I would be allowed to go home. *Home.* The word waltzed joyously across my tongue. Marc was planning to pick me up after work on Friday.

I worked very hard that week with my new team. This was the last "leg" of my hospital tour where I would learn to walk again. I was determined to progress quickly so I could get home, not just for a visit, but to stay.

When my physiotherapist asked if I wanted to walk on my knees I responded in the affirmative without hesitation.

She navigated the movements step-by-step with her own body, attempting to determine if I could do it with mine.

Once she was done, she positioned a mat on the floor at the foot of the bench. I slid onto my belly, then over the edge and onto the mat.

With all my weight on my knees, and no feet to balance me, I shuffled sideways along the edge of the bench. My muscles trembled and my heart pounded. Pain radiated from my knees, and beneath the gauze-like bandages on my thigh my skin stretched to its limit, but I pressed on.

When I returned to my room and the nurse unwrapped my bandages, my heart dropped. The site was clearly infected and turning purple and black in spots. *Is the flesh eating coming back?* The doctors responded by putting me on antibiotics. I had heard that amputees walk through pain every day. The faces of my children flashing through my mind reminded me that I was ready to do the same.

As they rolled me through the halls, I noticed there were many young people on the ward. Mostly men. At this hospital, I was in a section designed specifically for amputees. Everyone else was missing at least one limb, some two.

My occupational therapist concentrated on attempting to desensitize my arms. After I transferred to the bench, she set buckets filled with soft tissues, pebbles, shavings of iron bits, and gravel-like substances beside me. She asked me to repeatedly rub the ends of my arms in the various materials in order to desensitize them, as sometimes residual limbs can be over-sensitive. This would prepare my limbs for the pressure caused by wearing prosthetics. A full-length mirror was set up to one side of me, and she walked over and wheeled it farther away.

Over the next few days, she placed me on a disc-like cushion and had me move beanbags from one side of the bench to the other. The two-inch-high disc was designed to test the limits of my balance.

"If you like, I can move the mirror over and you can see how strong your balance is." She gestured to the mirror on the other side of the gym. "But only if you are comfortable."

Is she concerned I will be uncomfortable with what I see?

She waited for me to agree before bringing the mirror over and setting it up in front of me.

Slowly and cautiously, I raised my eyes to look at my reflection. Until now I had only seen my face in a mirror. I studied my missing hands and feet. My stumps ended where my calves would have been. They dangled off the side of the gym bench much like a child's feet hanging off the edge of a stool. My gaze travelled slowly up to my arms, which ended just below my elbows. Raising my eyes a little more, I let them settle on my face. Although my hair was much thinner, my face appeared relatively the same as the last time I had seen it. The hollow appearance in my eyes had softened a bit.

A voice from inside taunted, *How could anyone love this?* I lifted my chin, peering down my nose at my shimmering legs while I pushed the voice away.

This was the new me; I was alive, and God would get me home to my children.

19

"Sing to the LORD a new song, for he has done marvellous things..."

—Psalm 98:1

THE CITY LANDSCAPE TURNED TO ONE OF TREES AND GENTLE HILLS AS we entered suburbia. I told Marc all about my week as he drove me home, focusing on the things that seemed almost normal. The blur of green pastures streaming past the window brought a longing for my previous life.

I attempted a chuckle as I sat in the front seat with no feet, stumps dangling in the air. I braced myself with an arm on the door frame for extra security.

Marc checked over his shoulder as he pulled into the left turn lane. "I asked the nanny to prepare dinner for us tonight before she leaves." We turned and continued up a road that was twenty minutes from our home. "Tomorrow Chris and Deanna are coming to visit with their daughters, and Sunday we're going to church."

My stomach flipped. *I had to meet more new people?* I'd spent my week getting to know my new care team. My head was spinning. How would they react when they saw me?

Why is he going to church now? How many times had I asked Marc if we could go to church, and he would always find an excuse? Now *he* had chosen the church. My stomach knotted and I leaned forward in the seat.

Marc glanced over at me. As if he could read my thoughts, he said, "Don't worry, they are really nice people and the sermons are great. They've been praying for you and will be excited to meet you." He turned his gaze back to the road.

A memory of the kindly pastor and his wife who had visited me flashed through my mind. The strawberry milkshake they had brought me was the first thing I had been able to taste and enjoy.

Where had Marc's new-found love for God come from? How many times had I wished he could just have faith that God would pull us through? Through the adoption, our marriage, Liam's conception, I had never witnessed faith in him before.

When we pulled into the driveway, Cienna was waiting and jumping up and down. The sight of the nanny holding Liam in her arms jabbed at my heart, but I successfully pushed the resentment away. Because I couldn't get up and run to her, I hugged my daughter from the seat of the car.

Heat crept up my neck as Marc carried me into the house. I worried that the neighbours would see me. But again, I pushed the feeling away.

I also shoved back the thought of what it would be like to have to ask my mom to take me to the washroom. I tried not to think about the fact that, because I didn't have legs, I couldn't get up to use a toilet in the night, so someone had positioned a chair called a commode beside my bed for me to use.

I ignored the sense of lost dignity that swirled around me, and everything else that was out of my control. I focused on our children.

When it was bedtime, Marc carried me into Cienna's bedroom and I read her all of our favourite stories. I also told her some new ones that I had written in my head while lying immobile in the hospital.

"Don't go until I fall asleep, okay Mommy?" Her eyelids were getting heavy. She turned onto her side. "Can you rub my back?"

I reached out and gently rubbed Ren along her back until she nodded off. Then I called Marc and he picked me up, carried me across the hall, and carefully placed me in bed. How soothing it was to be in my own, comfortable bed.

Marc had nestled Liam between us. "I am so happy to have you home." He caressed my cheek.

Before long he rolled over and fell asleep. The purring sound of both my boys softly snoring warmed my heart.

I slipped the end of my arm into Liam's hand, trying not to disturb him. His little baby fingers clasped Stumpy.

God, thank you for letting me live.

In those moments, those tiny precious moments, I was a mom again.

❁ ❁ ❁

In the night Liam awoke, crying. Every time I attempted to console him he pushed me away. He only responded to Marc. I was devastated, but all the more determined to win him over.

We were thrilled to welcome Chris and Deanna and their girls for a visit the next morning. When Marc decided to go out and run an errand, they offered to watch the kids and stay with me. Liam was inconsolable. The only person he would allow to feed him was Chris, until Marc arrived back home. My heart ached in deep, unreachable places. *God, help my son to remember me. Help me to be patient as I wait.*

When Marc carried me to bed that night, after our friends had served us dinner and departed for their home, I contemplated how the weekend had gone. Tomorrow afternoon, following church and lunch, Marc would take me back to the hospital. I had made little progress with Liam. *God, how long will it take for him to know me?*

By the time Marc carried me to the car and loaded up the wheelchair the next morning, we were all exhausted. We pulled into the church parking lot and sat there for what seemed like several minutes.

Finally, Marc pushed open the car door and climbed out. He lifted me into the wheelchair and Cienna pushed me as he carried Liam and we entered the doors of the church. My stomach was churning. Another new experience. *I am tired of new experiences.*

My gaze caught some familiar faces; Cienna's teacher greeted me with a hug, and introductions happened all around us. The kind pastor and his wife also welcomed me. A gentleman pointed to a row that had room for my chair. The service started as we took our seats. Warmth travelled up my face as I noticed my name was on the board for prayer.

As everyone started singing a praise song, I looked at Marc. He was smiling and singing loudly. He got so little sleep, had so much to carry, including me. That should have frustrated him, but there he was, grinning broadly, obviously very much at home. The Marc I had married was so different from this man.

I opened my mouth and joined in the singing. My heart felt at home here too.

20

"You will be secure, because there is hope; you will look about you and take your rest in safety."

—Job 11:18

THE ROAD INTO THE REHABILITATION HOSPITAL HAS MANY TURNS. Each turn displays a sign pointing the driver in the right direction. Marc was taking me back to the hospital. At each turn my stomach rolled just a little bit more. As I neared the place that represented my current situation, I fought back the assailing thought, *This is not what my life is supposed to be.*

It was in those gut-wrenching, heartbreaking moments that this new life became inconceivable. It was in those moments that the attacks came strong and furious. I prayed for God to help me steel myself against the wave of emotions threatening to drown me. A mixture of longing, fear, anxiety, and homesickness simmered in my soul. *I will not let my family see me cry. I will prepare myself for that moment when they leave me at the hospital for the week. I will focus on getting through to next weekend, when I can go home to my family again.*

My first weekend at home reminded me of the challenges I faced. Regardless of the precious moments I had with my son, Liam continuously pushed me away. His bonds were to Marc and the nanny.

Focus on the tiny precious moments of motherhood, came from somewhere inside.

The joy on my daughter's face over just being with me helped ease the pain. *Enjoy these moments.* The voice echoed in my head ... or was it my heart?

I whispered to myself, "Focus on the joy in your heart as you sang at church this morning."

As we rolled to the room, a young lady I had seen in the gym on Friday wheeled toward us. Her left leg rested on the "stump board" of her wheelchair, wrapped in a bandage like mine.

"Look, Mommy, she has a leg just like yours!" Cienna jabbed the air with her finger as she pointed.

The woman smiled as she reached us. "Hi, I'm Heather."

I introduced my family and we continued to my hospital room. I was glad my daughter had seen Heather. It would help her, as it had me, to know that I was not the only person who had lost limbs, that there were others just like me.

They stayed with me for a few minutes while I transferred into my bed. I listened to their voices growing fainter as they travelled back down the hallway, then I put on a movie. I would not cry tonight.

※ ※ ※

It didn't take long to get into a regular routine. Every morning breakfast would arrive at 8:30 and then I waited for one of the nurses to come help me get dressed. When I was ready, I had an appointment in the gym where I would work on exercises that strengthened my muscles, often repetitions of leg or arm lifts at various angles. It felt good to be working out. The gym was always busy with several patients and their physical therapists or rehab assistants. Numerous parallel bars assisted with walking, and padded tables were set up around the room for patients to transfer onto and commence exercising.

After several rounds of many leg and arms lifts, I headed back upstairs for lunch, where my parents sometimes joined me. After lunch, I had an occupational therapy appointment. There I performed actions such as throwing beanbags into buckets on the floor in front of me. I quickly realized that throwing the beanbags took great strength and concentration. I sat on the edge of a bench and, as I grabbed the bags, I tried to pick up momentum with each swing of my arms. I pitched many bags near the bucket and some even landed inside. *Will this come in handy when I'm playing basketball with my kids one day?*

I was re-learning every task, as if I were a newborn. I smiled, thinking of my little boy and how we were learning together. If I tried to attempt an action at the same angle or in the same way that I would've done it before I got sick, I would fail. Failing meant that darkness would try to creep into my heart again.

My new electric wheelchair arrived, so once I passed the driving test I would be able to drive myself around. My therapists had ordered a chair with a joy stick to control the steering and mobility. The stick was installed at the precise angle for my stumps to reach it. Various pylons were placed on the gym floor in an obstacle course, zigzag pattern. I was instructed to weave in and out of them with the chair. Heather and I had been talking and were quickly becoming friends. She came down to the gym for her appointment with another patient, an older gentleman named Bryan. Bryan had lost both legs below the knee due to diabetes. He had sparkling blue eyes, white hair, and the most loving smile I had ever seen. Trying to weave my way around the path, I knocked over a pylon. All eyes in the gym were on me, and my face warmed.

"You just killed a Chihuahua." Heather laughed. Bryan's twinkly blue eyes joined her in laughter, and before I could think about it, I was laughing too.

"Watch out for those Chihuahuas!" Bryan joked.

It felt good to laugh. How long had it been?

We made our way down the halls and back upstairs to the amputee wing. "I've been trying to convince Cienna that I spend my weeks here training to be a superhero." The elevator doors opened. "But she won't believe me."

"Would she believe you if we showed up at your door one day in Superman outfits?" Bryan chuckled.

"Thanks Bryan, the image of you in blue tights is something I'm not going to be able to get out of my head." I shook my head, giggling. I was surfacing, the old me coming up for air.

Later as I was watching a movie on my iPad, Heather rolled into my room, eyes shining. "They're sending me home!"

"That's great!" I tried hard to sound like I meant it. I had been at this rehab hospital for three weeks, and I still didn't have my legs. The system was starting to frustrate me. In the real world, I could go to the gym whenever I felt like it or had time. I could control my level of fitness. Here, I had no control. I had to wait for the care team to decide when it was time for me to receive my new legs. I had been waiting for several weeks, and I thought by now I would have them. The desire to get home and on with my life was growing greater and greater. Yet I was at a standstill. The frustration fought to rise up within me and it was becoming harder to swallow it down.

21

"Now faith is confidence in what we hope for and assurance about what we do not see."

—Hebrews 11:1

WHEN MY DOCTOR CAME IN AND ANNOUNCED, "WE'RE GOING TO START making your arms. You'll be casted this week," I was thrilled.

They had planned to start with my legs, but I'd continued to struggle with infections in the donor site where they had removed skin.

The specialists who ordered my prosthetics had strange and unfamiliar titles. No matter how many times I tried, I couldn't remember what I was expected to call them. All the doctors' names and their positions were posted at the nurses' station outside my room, so I drove my wheelchair there. Physiatrist. I tried to roll the word around in my mind. It sounded like psychiatrist to me, and I couldn't quite pronounce the difference. My physiatrist wrote a prescription for my prosthetics, and my prosthetist was responsible for filling that prescription by designing and creating my prosthetics.

To make a cast, my prosthetist put a bucket in front of him and, while he sat in front of me, dropped a toilet paper-sized roll of mesh-like white material into the bucket. Once wet, the material became a pliable plaster that he wrapped around the ends of my arms. The cast would be used to make a socket, a piece of plastic that my arms would fit into. The socket would be attached to a metal hook. Wires would run from the metal hooks, along my arms, to the back of my shoulders. Spreading my arms put stress on the wires and opened up the hooks. When I relaxed my shoulders, the hooks would also relax and close.

In a few days, I was sitting back in front of my prosthetist, inserting my stumps into the new arms. Nothing could have prepared me for the mixed emotions that accosted me when I gazed down to see my hands were now two metal hooks. *Once again, I'm faced with the loss of my femininity.* Loss crept up on me as I thought of my fingers and nails. I sighed heavily, and pushed back on the wave. *They will help me to do more, like feeding Liam.*

When I wheeled back to the ward with my new hooks on, Heather and Bryan were waiting for me in the doorway to my room. I was excited to see them.

"See if you can pick that up." Heather pointed to the tray of water bottles that had been set on the floor outside my room, waiting to be distributed. I tried to place the hooks into the handle on the large water bottle. I was able to get them through on the first try, but the angle at which I would lift the water bottle to my mouth seemed off and I let it go.

"Let's go for lunch." Bryan headed through the ward and downstairs to the cafeteria. I studied my arms as I followed him. The new prosthetics seemed so clumsy and awkward.

We sat at the picnic tables outside, listening to the birds singing.

"Let's see if you can open up the ketchup packet with your new hands." Heather nodded at the packets, encouraging me.

I took a deep breath and lifted up a packet. It required great concentration, but I managed to get both hooks clasped upon it. My tongue stuck out the corner of my mouth as I tried to tear away a section of the ketchup package. The plastic simply slipped over the surface of the hooks. There was not enough tension. The harder I tried, the more difficult the task grew. I resisted the urge to toss the packet across the lawn. How did I open ketchup before?

I smiled and opened it with my teeth. The exact same way I would have opened it if I had hands. We all laughed at the irony.

Over the next few days, I worked at overcoming the thought that the appearance of the hooks robbed me of femininity. I planned what I would do with them when I arrived home. To Liam, I was still that strange lady who came to visit on weekends, so the first thing I did when I went into the house was to use them to feed him.

Sitting in my wheelchair in front of his high chair, I moved my shoulders to open the pincers and grab hold of the plastic yellow baby spoon. I released them to allow them to clamp on, but missed. I pushed the spoon around on the tray, trying to place it at the perfect angle. After a few attempts, I was able to clamp on. I lifted my arm from the shoulder, instead of bending my elbow, so that I could carefully dip the spoon into the glass jar of food. Then, making sure it was at the right angle, I maneuvered it into his mouth. He cooed and waved his hands, anxious for more food. I had hoped for a sense of connectedness, a held gaze, or a twinkle in his eye. There was none. *I am the stranger who visits on the weekend.* I concentrated on carefully feeding him. *God, how long will it take him to know me?*

Later that afternoon, I watched Cienna playing in front of the TV and had an idea. "Cienna, grab some nail polish!"

She skipped to her room. When she returned, she held a beautiful, bright-pink polish. She grinned as she handed it to me. Glancing at the cap, I realized I would not be able to remove it with my claws. Instead of twisting the top off, I clenched my teeth around the cap and twisted it open using my arms. It was opposite to how I would have opened it with hands, but it worked.

"Can you hold the bottle for me?" Her strong, six-year-old fingers wrapped around it, and I lifted out the applicator brush. "You can set it down now." She placed the bottle on the table in front of us. I pointed to my thigh. "Place your hand here and keep it flat."

Holding my breath, I carefully brushed her first finger nail. Each stroke represented another step closer to being the mom that I used to be.

When I finished, Cienna looked at me, her brown eyes sparkling. "You did it, Mommy. You painted my nails."

I *had* done it. Flushed with victory, I held up the brush. "Let's do your toenails too!"

22

"...but those who trust in the Lord will find new strength. They will soar high on wings like eagles. They will run and not grow weary. They will walk and not faint."

—Isaiah 40:31

EVERY MOTHER REMEMBERS HOW OLD HER CHILD WAS WHEN HE OR SHE first walked. My daughter was seventeen months old, one month short of having to walk down the aisle as a flower girl. At nine months, Liam was not yet able to walk, so he still held onto furniture as he tried to wobble between the table and the couch. I had been hospitalized for almost five months when my new, prosthetic legs were finally ready to go on. I would stand for the first time today.

Unless you're standing, your body is never in a straight position. My care team had worked hard to ensure that the muscles in my core and legs would be strong enough to support me. I smiled all the way through the hallways of my ward, down the elevators, and past the main lobby to the fitting room. But inside I was praying, just as I had been for many weeks.

God, I know that prosthetics hurt. Please give me the strength and endurance that I need to walk again. I am scared. Please God, let me walk again. Let me get my life back.

I maneuvered my chair between two parallel bars and couldn't help but laugh to myself. All new amputees learning to walk started by clutching the bars and bracing themselves while trying to take their first steps. Had anyone considered the fact that I wouldn't be able to hold on to them?

Henry sat in front of me with a set of prosthetic legs that had been casted to fit my remaining limbs. A therapist hovered on each side of me, the two women who had been helping to prepare me physically for this moment. Marc had arranged to be there as well and greeted me with a great big smile and warm, loving eyes.

My new legs were made of long, cylindrical metal poles that connected to a carbon blade. The blade sat inside a foot shell. The feet had a pair of white laced-up running shoes on them.

"Okay, let's see how they feel." My prosthetist rolled a long silicone liner onto the end of my leg. This would be a buffer between the socket and my delicate skin. As if slipping my feet into a brand new pair of heels, I carefully slid my stumps into the sockets. I was locked in once they rolled the liners and sleeves to the tops of my thighs.

I was ready to go. Butterflies fluttered in my stomach as I slid to the edge of my seat. As I prepared to stand between the bars, the women stabilized me by putting their hands under my arms.

I tried to stand up, but I didn't get very far. I couldn't seem to push myself up high enough. "I think I need to put my elbows into the palms of your hands."

I dug my elbows deep into their palms.

"Keep going!" Henry cheered as I pushed hard, lifting myself up with my elbows.

It was difficult and took great strength, but I was almost there. I dug deeper with my elbows and pushed even harder, driven by the desire to walk.

I was standing.

But I wasn't straight.

"Keep going! You can lean on me if you have to, but keep going." My prosthetist braced my hips into a straight position.

I felt so supported with the women holding tightly onto my arms.

Like a roller coaster coming to a quick stop, my body seemed to click into position and I was standing up straight.

I let out a huge sigh of relief. When had I last taken a breath?

"Hey, you're standing!" Marc beamed with pride.

I caught a glimpse of myself in the mirror beside me. My hair and clothes were disheveled, and I didn't resemble the woman I had been five months ago, but I was standing. Ready to become the woman I was meant to be now. I smiled, shimmering legs and all. My heart danced with gratitude.

It wasn't long before Marc brought Cienna down to the hospital to see how I was getting around. Head high, I paraded around the room for her with my walker. I had only been moving around on my new legs for a few days.

The infectious giggle of my now six-year-old had everyone in the room smiling.

What a contrast to the previous weekend, when my heart had stopped for a moment, as if in failure again, at one sentence my daughter had spoken.

All the papers had been removed from the dining room table and we were all sitting down to dinner. Marc set a plate down in front of me. I still could not cut with my prosthetic arms, so he started slicing up my meat.

Everyone was chattering around the table. My dad was telling us about his day, and Liam was squealing and gurgling in his highchair.

A sad and disappointed voice echoed through the room. "Mom, prayers don't come true."

Everyone at the table stopped speaking and stared at Cienna.

My heart went on full alert. "What do you mean, sweetie?"

"I prayed for your legs to grow back and they didn't."

I froze. I dug deep inside to find something to say, but nothing came.

Yet here I was, upright on two legs in front of my girl. I crossed the room and leaned over the front of my walker to look her directly in the eye.

"See honey? Prayers do come true. Mommy got her legs back, didn't she?"

She smiled, a big, toothless smile that reflected in her eyes.

"Yes, Mama." She nodded, her eyes joyous as she jumped up from her chair to gently hug me.

It takes great concentration to walk on prosthetic legs. I spent days practicing in the hopes that I would hear the words, "You can go home now."

I wanted so badly to be able to go to the bathroom by myself, or even to just move around.

Discouragement tried to keep its stronghold on my by taunting me with the things I couldn't do, but I continued to push it away with faith that God was my enabler.

One day upon returning from the gym, I parked my electric wheelchair beside the bed. I was determined to walk unaided from my chair to my bed for the first time.

I reasoned that if I fell, it would be straight onto the bed.

As I had learned to do in every situation, I planned the movements I would need to make in my mind. *God, please lead me.* I would have to take two or three steps toward the bed, then turn around and sit down. My tray table was not too far from the bed, so if needed, I could lean my arm on it as I turned around.

With another prayer and a deep breath, I stood up.

My heart swelled. *I am standing all by myself.* The bed seemed to call to me, as though it had arms that reached out, ready to cradle me.

Oh please, God, don't let me fall.

It seemed so simple. Two or three steps and I would be on the bed. I bit my lip as I slid one leg ahead of the other. Soon I was turning around and had planted myself on the bed. I let out my breath in a rush. *I did it!*

Each day I practiced, walking farther and farther. First out the door of the room, then around the unit. With each step my heart cried out, *Take me home. Please, God, take me home.*

23

"The circle of love that lies upon my neck reflects the journey that brought me here. It confirms the steadfast love that was found along the way."

—Cyndi Desjardins Wilkens

I HAD JUST COME BACK FROM PHYSIOTHERAPY AND WAS RESTING IN THE hospital bed when Heather dropped by for a visit.

"The doctor said I can go home in a week." I straightened up. "Marc wants me to plan a vacation by the beach."

She sat down on the chair beside me. "Oh, nice. You can go swimming!"

"How?" I threw my arms up in exasperation. "I don't have swim legs. Marc would have to carry me into the water." I threw my body back down onto the bed, imagining all the people on the beach staring at me, openmouthed.

"'Look at that poor girl,' everyone will say." I glanced toward the hallway and lowered my voice. "It would be humiliating."

Heather raised an eyebrow. "People will be looking at you in envy. Can you imagine how romantic it would be?" Her eyes sparkled as she leaned forward. "How many women wish their husbands would do that for them?"

"Heather, you always see the positive in everything." I rested my arm across my chest, imagining the wedding ring that used to be on my finger. A circle of love.

I was going home for the weekend of our eleventh wedding anniversary. I had no idea if I would get something from Marc. I had browsed around the shops and hospital vendors, but nothing seemed to speak to me.

After his long weeks, he was tired on the weekends. Fortunately, my mother was there to help me with any undignified needs such as toileting. However, it was Marc who had to lift me up and carry me from room to room. It was Marc who picked me up at the hospital every Friday and dropped me off every Monday morning.

Was I a burden? I worried that this was too much for him to carry. I had to fight that feeling or it would take me away, lifting me like a kite in the wind. Up and up and then snagging on a tree branch, unable to fly.

A small gift bag waited for me in the car. "Happy Anniversary, honey!"

"But I didn't get you anything." I contemplated the bag. It was light blue with gold letters. Jewelry.

"That's okay." Reaching his hand into the bag, Marc pulled out a small box. "I'll open it for you."

Inside the box lay a gold chain with my wedding and engagement rings on it.

"When you were sick, I took your rings and put them on my chain with my cross." He opened the clasp and motioned for me to bend forward so he could fasten it around my neck.

As we drove home I studied my husband. I had woken up from the coma to a different man. It was as if he had been transformed into the husband I had always dreamed of.

At some point along this journey, he had found God. Or, to be more accurate, somewhere through it all God had found him.

How I would have loved to have heard his conversations with God.

I looked back out the window at the rolling hills that led to our suburban neighbourhood. Who was this man God had given me?

24

"Search me, God, and know my heart; test me and know my anxious thoughts. See if there is any offensive way in me, and lead me in the way everlasting."

—Psalm 139:23-24

FROM MY VANTAGE POINT, PROPPED AGAINST THE PILLOWS, I WATCHED my nurse as she prepared me for the night. By the end of the week I would be home. I'd grown used to the nurse brushing my teeth and hair and helping me get ready to sleep. Although I had learned so much, I still could not dress myself. *What would it be like trying to manage at home?*

I thought back over my journey. For almost six months I had worked very hard to become well enough to go home. They had predicted it would take a year of hospital rehabilitation before I could return to my life. Now my dream was coming true. My prayers were being answered.

I chuckled, remembering the many times I'd had to place rings on poles or throw beanbags across the room, so many silly little games that seemed to have no point at all, but worked toward making me stronger and more agile.

I had received a phone call from Bev earlier in the week. "A national television network wants to do an interview with you." She forwarded the information to Marc and me. We set up the interview for Friday, first at the hospital and then later, at home, where additional footage would be shot.

Fear was starting to set in. The idea of so many people seeing me on television with no hands made me want to run screaming from my room. Would they judge me? Would they think that, somehow, I deserved what had happened to me? I frowned. Why would I even think something like that? Deep down, was I still holding on to the notion that all of this was the result of something I had done wrong? Surely I had let that go. *What if people think I'm ugly with no hands and feet?* The nervousness in my stomach was developing into full-blown nausea.

God, I'm not sure I can do this. I really don't want people to see me like this.

A movement at the sink across the room caught my eye, bringing me back to the present. My nurse had hesitated a moment before turning and walking toward me, clutching my toothbrush in her hand. "You know, Cyndi, sometimes God uses us as messengers."

There it was. The answer to my *why?* Somewhere deep inside my heart I had known it. I was just like the bleeding woman, but I had spent my life searching for other things to place my faith in. Now, in my second chance at life, my faith rested in Jesus. If God needed me to be his messenger, my soul would rejoice in that purpose.

25

> "The LORD is close to the broken hearted and saves those who are crushed in spirit."
>
> —Psalm 34:18

A GARDENER DOESN'T JUST PLANT A SEED AND EXPECT IT TO GROW. HE takes time to plan out what is best for his particular seeds. Cultivated soil must be a good mix of loose, fertile ground. The seed must be planted at just the right spot for optimal growth. That seed then requires the perfect amount of sun and rain. If there's too much rain, the seed could wash away. If there is too much sun, the plant could become scorched. The mix of fertile ground, the right amount of sun and light, and an adequate amount of rain, will ensure a successful harvest.

However, there are many things that can uproot a planted seed. Birds or other predators can eat it up. If the soil is not of good quality, if it is uncultivated or rocky, the seed cannot take root. Harsh weather can stunt growth or destroy the growing plant.

The seeds of hope and faith that had been planted in my heart, perhaps when I was born, perhaps during those many times I sat holding my white, leather-bound Bible, had strengthened me. My faith had been buffeted by a torrential downpour, but it had also experienced sunlight and love.

And so I continued to grow.

✳ ✳ ✳

One late-summer morning, the sun crept slowly up over the tops of the trees in our suburban neighbourhood. I had just slipped my legs on and was creeping down the hallway. Everyone was still asleep, and I was trying not to wake them, a difficult task with prosthetic feet. With no ankle, I was unable to tiptoe. Each step caused the hardwood floor to creak a little bit, but I had learned to minimize the weight of my foot in a way that also minimized the noise.

Early morning was one of my favourite times of the day. I would sit at our table in the solarium-like room just off the kitchen, where floor-to-ceiling windows allowed light to stream through in the morning. As the sun rose, God's love warmed me.

My Bible rested on the table in front of me. I had been spending my mornings reading it. Scripture was speaking to the very heart of my life. Perhaps it had been locked in my heart all along and I simply needed to open the treasure chest. Why hadn't I done so before? As I read through the pages, I found the answers to questions that resided within my soul.

On those mornings, my soul was refreshed. It needed to be refreshed, because every day it seemed as though my spirit would be squashed just that little bit more. But here, in the sunlight of the early morning, with the Word of the One who had pulled me through, that spirit was renewed and I would be ready to take on the fight of the day.

I thought the journey would get easier once I came home from the hospital, like an Olympic medalist after finishing her race. But the marathon had only begun. Battles broke out on numerous fronts. Every day I tried to learn new things and attempt new activities. Everything took much longer to do than it had before I got sick, and required an incredible amount of planning.

But there was a battle that far surpassed the physical battle I was in. There was a battle of spirit. Jesus was now my hands and feet. I felt armed and ready to take on that battle.

When I first arrived home from the hospital in July, I was unable to dress myself or put on my prosthetics. In the morning I stayed in bed, waiting for my personal support worker to arrive and assist me. By that time Marc would have rolled out of bed and headed off to work, after kissing me lightly on the forehead and wishing me a good day. Morning sounds, the music of the household, surrounded me: Liam waking up and making little baby noises for the nanny, or Cienna running down the hallway and into the kitchen for breakfast before heading to school. The sounds were the same as the ones I'd heard in the past, but now they seemed so different, because I could not respond to them. I could not be there, in those moments. *Will life ever return to normal?*

Music can bring joy or sadness. It was in those moments, while listening to the music of my home, that I reflected upon the mother that I had been, and prayed for God to help me to become the mother I wanted to be again.

Slowly I started moving around the house, getting my footing on prosthetic legs. I spent my days trying to reach out to Liam and being with Cienna after school. I had many conversations with God, asking Him to show Liam who I was.

One hot summer evening as I lay resting, the nanny came into my bedroom and placed my son on my lap. He was dressed in his little red and white striped onesie, and although he fussed when she left, I was able to settle him. I put *Veggie Tales* on the television, stroking his head and face with my bare stumps as I tried to get him to fall asleep. My heart nearly jumped out of my chest with joy as he snuggled into me and started to drowse off. I was afraid that my heart was pounding so loudly it would wake him and put an end to this very precious moment.

The ringing of the phone jolted him awake. Before I could settle him back down, the nanny, having finished her five-minute shower, rushed in to respond to his cries. She lifted him up and took him away. But lying in bed that night, staring out the window, I focused on that moment he nestled into my bosom. The moment my heart felt as if it was going to beat right out of my chest. I clung to that memory and dreamt of the day he would know me as his mom.

❋ ❋ ❋

In the evenings, I would ask Marc to walk with me. As a family, we ventured farther and farther around the block with Marc holding my right arm.

One humid August afternoon as I sat on the couch and watched Liam and Cienna playing in front of the television, I was overwhelmed with thoughts of the tasks I couldn't do. *Everything in my home is out of reach.*

How long before I can make dinner, brush Cienna's hair, make her lunch? I shifted my position on the couch. I wanted to be a participant in my life, not just an observer.

"Let's go to the park." I dug my stump into the arm of the couch and pushed myself up. On the way to my wheelchair, I picked up the remote and fumbled to turn the TV off. Somehow, I hit the power button.

The park was not far from our home, but I wasn't strong enough to try to walk there alone. I had walked short distances around the outside of the house, but was unsure of taking such a big step so soon. The children were thrilled, though, so as we prepared, I asked the nanny to join us.

The cool breeze on my face, even from a wheelchair, revived me. "Are you excited to go on vacation next week?" I asked Cienna.

"Yes!" She skipped along the tree-lined pathway.

"Remember how we loved to look for frogs?"

She nodded.

"Let's see if we can find any." I was a bit relieved when we didn't, as I wasn't sure how I could possibly pick one up.

As we came to the park, I was thankful to see that no one else was there. I kept my eyes on the children as they played, and even rolled my chair over to push Liam in his baby swing. I was able to get up and move around a bit, although the wood chips on the playground made me feel as though I was walking on a trampoline—wobbly and unstable.

As I watched the children having fun, I glanced up at the sky. *Please, Lord, let me be able play with them here one day.*

A young boy of around eight arrived at the park. His eyes were fixed on me, sitting in my wheelchair with hook-like arms and metal legs. I knew he wanted to ask me questions, so I waited for him to approach.

"What happened to your arms?" Before I could say anything, Cienna responded. "My mom got sick, but God let her live. They had to amputate her feet, so now she has prosthetics." Her six-year-old voice sounded mat-ter-of-fact as she spoke the big words. I smiled to myself.

My gaze travelled to Liam. He was now ten months old and just learn-ing to walk by holding onto the nanny's hands. She led him up the small baby slide and gave him a little nudge down. When he reached the bottom, he fell and scraped his knee. I wanted to jump out of my wheelchair, pick him up, and hold him close, as a mother does with her wounded child. But he immediately ran to the nanny, looking at her as though *she* was his mother. What worried me even more, though, deep within my soul, was the fact that she looked at him as though she was his mother as well. Unable to bear it, I turned my face away, resolving within my heart to find ways to show him who I was.

※ ※ ※

A week later I found myself sitting beside a campfire, staring up at the starry night. We were on our first vacation since my stay in the hospital.

As I watched the clouds moving slowly in to cover the stars, I noticed that one star, just to the right of the moon, remained exposed.

I hadn't been prepared for the longings that accosted me on this vacation. This was our third and final night at the resort. Everywhere I turned, I was reminded of what I had done on previous vacations. I told myself I was blessed to have those memories. What if they had been lost as well?

Marc continued to amaze me. I was still trying to process the difference I saw in this man and I shook my head, astounded, every time I came to the four steps up onto the deck and he rushed over and carried me up.

On the first day of our vacation, we had been able to drive our van onto the beach. Marc pulled out several lawn chairs and placed them alongside the rolling waves of the water. I watched him as he removed his T-shirt, scooped up Liam, and beckoned Cienna to follow him into the lake. The waves were high, and the children squealed with delight. The memories of the beaches I had visited in my life came upon me like waves.

God, how could you take this from me too? You know I love the beach. I turned my face away as tears welled in my eyes. Visions of my feet buried in soft sand, and of me, running along the beach holding hands with my daughter, came crashing in on me, and I felt as though I was drowning in memories.

"Let's go for a walk on the beach." Marc stood over me, dripping wet and drawing me back to the present. He slid his arms under my elbows and helped lift me up out of my chair. We strolled on the beach without speaking as he held onto the hook where my hand would have been. Slowly he moved his hand up to my shoulder. We walked along the edge of the waves for quite some time. Liam stayed behind with the nanny, and Cienna trailed behind us, picking up shells and rocks along the way.

Words strayed from my mouth before I could stop them. Words that I had held inside my heart for fear others would think I was ungrateful for the life God had given me.

"I don't understand why God would take the beach away from me too." As soon as I heard myself say the words, I regretted them.

Marc stopped and faced me. "Oh honey, think about it, this is only temporary. One day we will get you legs to swim with, and you'll be back in the water."

He was right. It was far too soon for me to be able to get swim legs; the wounds from my surgeries still bled at night when I removed my prosthetics.

I looked down the sand; his bare footprints and my prosthetic foot-prints were displayed side by side. I smiled as I pointed them out to him. "It's similar to this life; it's only temporary, a small part of the life we will have one day in heaven."

The second day brought an even hotter sun. After hours in the heat at the beach, we strolled along the boardwalk. Marc walked beside me with Cienna, and the nanny followed with the stroller and Liam. My prosthetic arms were unbearably hot and heavy. The plastic was suffocating, and the insides of my sockets were drenched in sweat.

Marc noticed my discomfort. "Why don't you take them off?"

I had never been seen without them in public, but I removed them and stored them in the bottom of the stroller.

As I studied the stroller, I took a breath of courage. *Why can't I push it?* I positioned my forearms on the bar of the stroller handle where I would have gripped it with my hands before. I cautiously pushed, trying to ease my way through the busy promenade. I was so focused on what I was doing that I barely noticed the number of people watching me.

I turned to Marc. "I guess this makes me a hands-on mom again!" I smiled.

❄ ❄ ❄

My brother-in-law decided to bring his two daughters and son down to visit us at the cabin. We had gotten caught in the rain earlier, so I took my legs off and lounged on the couch. It felt good to remove the many layers of plastic and silicone that had baked my stumps like loaves of bread in the heat.

Once again, I felt like a spectator as everyone else enjoyed a conversation. The nanny had set watermelon out for everyone to grab. I caught a glimpse of her in the kitchen, feeding some to Liam. He was eating it fast and she was giggling at him. Before I could tell her he was too young for it, I noticed that Liam seemed to be choking. The last piece of watermelon she had given him must have gotten stuck in his throat. I sat up.

"He's choking!" My scream echoed through the cabin.

Marc ran to Liam.

I pressed my stumps together as in prayer. "Please God, let him be okay." My eyes met my niece's, and I could see her empathy for me reflected in them. Marc had turned our son over on his hand and was patting his back. A large piece of watermelon flew from his mouth.

While Liam was choking, I was reminded of everything I had lost. But as soon as he coughed up the watermelon, I was reminded of everything I had gained.

It was in that moment of helplessness that I realized that I needed Jesus. I needed Him to hold my hand in every parenting moment. There was no way I could do this on my own. If Marc had not gotten to Liam as fast as he had …

Every time I watched my children on the monkey bars, every fall they took, I would need Jesus holding my hand. I couldn't jump up and save my children. I wasn't ready to do it all on my own. Perhaps I would never be. I needed Him.

That last night, sitting around the fire, my eyes were drawn back to the night sky and that one, exiled star. The loneliness that had haunted me throughout our marriage was gone. My husband was a different man. Perhaps I had changed as well. I struggled with a different loneliness now, one that, if I allowed it to seep in, could easily place my heart in exile. It was a loneliness steeped in the knowledge that this walk I took on prosthetic legs

I had to take by myself. I was surrounded by loving friends and family, but none of them could know or truly understand how I felt. The exiled star reminded me of the words I had read over and over again in the Bible, *I will never leave you nor forsake you.*

For several months, I had been immobile in the hospital. It was there that Jesus had reached out His hand and touched me—the woman no one else wanted to touch—with words from His book.

"I knit you together in your mother's womb. You were fearfully and wonderfully made." I was not in exile. I wasn't walking by myself. God was with me. He truly knew what each step meant, and He would not leave me to take a single one of them alone.

26

> "Trust in the LORD with all your heart and lean not on
> your own understanding; in all your ways submit to
> him, and he will make your paths straight."
>
> —Proverbs 3:5-6

THE DOORBELL RANG AND CIENNA RAN TO ANSWER IT. I KNEW WHO
it was, and waited for her reaction. Her squeals of joy filled the foyer as I
walked to the front door to find my friends, Bryan and Heather, dressed as
Superman and Supergirl. They had also dressed up Heather's dog in his superhero costume. "We are here for your mom!" They struggled to maintain
their serious faces. "We have crime to fight!"

As they walked in the door, Cienna protested, "Mom is not a superhero; she doesn't have any superpowers!"

"Yes, she does," Heather laughed as she walked across the foyer and
into our living room. "She has the power of inspiration!" She sat down on
the couch beside me. "How are you doing?" I noted Bryan's fatigue as he
sank onto the chair across from me. It had been difficult going up the front
steps of my house, but he was smiling.

"You can see I don't bump from wall-to-wall like a Weeble anymore."
I waved my arms to demonstrate that I was walking without any walking
aids. I had become stronger and stronger on my new legs. In the beginning,
I would bump around, joking that I was one of those little pear-shaped
figurines that I had grown up with in the 70s, a Weeble that wobbled but
wouldn't fall down. Slowly, after a few months, I had learned to comfortably walk to and from the park with no walking aids except for Cienna or
Marc at my side.

"I picked up Liam." I smiled proudly. As I grew stronger, I longed for more motherhood moments such as changing a diaper, or picking up and holding my son. He was not yet walking, so he couldn't get away from me as fast as he might like. The other day, I had reached down to my twenty-pound child and, leaning back against the wall, picked him up and held him in my arms. It was a true milestone in my quest to be a "hands-on" mom again.

"I was thrilled, but my personal service worker walked in at that moment." My smile faded. "She looked horrified. She rushed over to take him from me, and said, 'You shouldn't pick him up! You might drop him!'"

The memory still stung. "I felt like a three-year-old child." Liam giggled from the kitchen where he was playing with the nanny. I adjusted the couch pillows behind my back. "None of these caregivers understand. I am young and have a family, and I have every intention of being a hands-on mother again." Cienna had joined Liam and the nanny and now both my children were giggling loudly. "It's like they want to put me in a box, and no matter what I do, I can't break out of it. They have an opinion of me, and I have to fight to change it."

Adrenaline coursed through me. Where was this strength of spirit coming from? One of the medical professionals I'd seen had said, "There is no medical explanation for you being alive right now." But I knew the explanation. And I knew the source. God had given me a spirit that far surpassed the strength of the human spirit.

Bryan chuckled, bringing me back to the present. "You mean you're *not* an elderly lady?" His blue eyes twinkled.

Heather leaned forward, clearly ready to continue the jest. She raised her voice so that Cienna could hear. "Bryan, she's a super hero, and we have crimes to fight!" Cienna came back into the room just as Heather stood up. "Let's get going to our crime fighter training sessions."

With that cue, Bryan slowly rose from the couch. "You're right, we better go."

My heart beat faster at the reminder of why he was there. He was taking me to my driving lesson. Bryan and Heather had driven an hour up from the city just to help me out. We put on our coats and walked out to the wheelchair van. Being amputees, none of us had to stop to put our shoes on.

While still at the hospital I had researched a rehabilitative driving facility. I was determined to get my license back.

I wasn't sure what to expect when we first walked into the facility. I was greeted by the owner, who was an occupational therapist. She took me into an office and put me through extensive testing to confirm that I had more than sufficient response in my right foot to drive.

She would notify the ministry that I was under her care when I retook my written test. I felt as though I was sixteen years old again, clutching my little booklet and preparing for the written—or in my case oral—exam.

It wasn't long before I found myself behind the wheel of the rehabilitative driving vehicle. As the therapist walked me through putting on my seatbelt, adjusting the mirrors, moving the seat, and ensuring that I could reach everything, I quickly calculated that I had been a licensed driver for twenty-seven years. My heart quickened. *I am about to do this all over again.* I was excited and ready. Then she pulled out a small bowl with a sheepskin lining. She inserted it into a clamp-like holder on the steering wheel. "This is a new product I found at a trade show. I think it might work for you, but you have to take both your arms off."

I glanced down at the hooks that continued to plague me. They prevented me from feeling my children's faces as I touched them and they seemed to attract so many open-mouthed stares from people. I took them off and set them on the floor, then placed my stump into the bowl on the steering wheel. It gave me great control.

As I maneuvered my way down the road, I felt as though I had never stopped driving. With the exception of having to turn my head a little farther to check my blind spot, and re-establishing the feel of my right foot touching the gas and brake, very little was different. I was behind the wheel again. One step closer to independence.

I could hardly wait to share the news with Marc. When we were all at the dinner table that evening, I reached for my glass and lifted it as though giving a toast. "I can drive with my right foot!"

His eyebrows raised and his mouth dropped open. "Really?" He was astounded as well. He shook his head, grinning. "How do you do it?"

I explained every detail as he listened intently.

When I finished, he stood up and walked to my side of the table and leaned over to kiss me. "You are my hero." My heart leapt.

As Marc cleared the dishes away, I couldn't stop smiling. Even the knowledge that it would take many months of practice before I was ready to test again couldn't take away from the thrill of that moment. I could drive.

After dinner, I took off my arms, determined to see what I could do without them. Lying in bed, my eyes were drawn to the back of the bedroom door where they were hanging.

I turned my head to look out my bedroom window at the night sky. *God, what if I am the only quadruple amputee driving? What if I am the first one?*

I rolled over on my side, placing my stumps under the pillow as I exhaled a sleepy sigh. *Did it matter?* God would carry me through. I put my complete trust in Him.

27

"Naked I came from my mother's womb, and naked I will depart. The Lord gave and the Lord has taken away; may the name of the Lord be praised."

—Job 1:21

FLOATING ON MY BACK IN THE DEEP END OF AN INDOOR POOL OF WARM salt water, I stretched a long, cat-like stretch from the tips of my missing toes right up to the ends of my imaginary fingernails.

I have always loved being in the water. The peaceful, relaxing act of floating lends itself to reflection. It is in those moments that I study the ceiling, willing my eyes past it and into the heavens. My heart overflows with gratefulness and I speak with God.

Thank you, God, for coming to my rescue and letting me live.

"See if you can hit 150 metres this time!" my physiotherapist cheered. I was treading water so I flipped onto my back. My pulse quickened. I was thrilled. In the water, everyone cheered me on. I simply had to look around the pool to see how astounded everyone was that I was swimming.

Thank you, God, for giving me back the gift of swimming.

As I started my strokes, I glanced over at my therapist and considered how far I'd come in learning to swim. I hadn't been home more than a month when my physiotherapist suggested I take rehabilitative swimming to strengthen my core. It was true; every movement I now took, such as walking up the stairs or ramps, or walking any distance, required great strength from the core of my body.

The rehab pool had a ledge on the side, which enabled me to sit down, remove my legs, and turn around to face the water. That first day when I sat at the edge of the pool, contemplating diving in, I felt naked. I was sure I heard gasps as people who were in the pool looked over and saw the scars all over my body, and my missing limbs. My dreams of bikini modelling came to an end in that moment.

As my physiotherapist beckoned for me to jump in that day, I scrutinized the water. I wasn't so sure. Although I had always loved swimming, now when I was in the water, I felt claustrophobic, and memories of being in a coma came back. Memories I couldn't call into sharp focus, but that filled me with the sensation of being held underwater and not allowed to come up for air.

It's not my first time in a pool. When I was still at the rehab hospital and coming home on weekends, Marc had tried to help me swim in our backyard pool. Lovingly, he outfitted me in a life jacket and the children's arm-floaties. I didn't have swim legs yet, so I would try to swim with just my stumps.

He gently lifted me over the edge of the pool and allowed me to slip in. I struggled to flip over onto my stomach. Marc jumped in and helped to roll me onto my back. As I tried to float around, my chest tightened. It was not the same as it has been before. I felt awkward, as though someone was pushing my head under the water and I couldn't stop it. I had no centre of buoyancy.

I had never been a good swimmer. I was very good at the doggy paddle, but since I needed hands for that, I wouldn't be competing in that category anytime soon.

That first day, doubts resurfaced. *I'm not sure I can do this.* In response, a voice I hadn't heard in quite some time came upon me. A still, small voice that came from inside, from my spirit. The spirit that had been nurtured with every scripture I had read. *If you had given into fear the first time you were asked to stand on your knees, to walk on your knees, or to walk on prosthetic legs, you wouldn't be here right now.*

I pushed back my shoulders. *I can do all things through Christ who strengthens me.* Those were words that had spoken to my heart many times throughout this journey. I took a deep breath and jumped into the water.

I was treated with loving care. My swim therapists started out by placing a paediatric blow-up ring around my neck. As a hit to my pride, and just to highlight that it was a children's ring, it had little rattles inside of it.

Every time I moved, it would jingle. But I was floating. Gently, patiently, my therapists guided me around the pool, and in no time, I was swimming.

"Who knew you could swim without hands and feet?" I'm sure my face glowed as I shared my experience with Marc that night.

"That's fifty metres." The voice of my swim therapist drew me back to the present. Lost in reminiscing, I had forgotten to count my laps.

Swimming brought me confidence and strength. Not just strength in my physical core, but strength in my resolve. This was good, because I would need that as I walked in the door to my home from a swimming lesson one afternoon.

Our nanny had a wide smile on her face as I removed my jacket. "He called me Mama today."

I stared at her. Was I hearing things? When I looked at her face, I knew. It was time to make a change.

I waited for Marc to come home and, when we were alone, I spoke up. "I think we need to find a new nanny." I shared the events of that day with my husband. Then, with some trepidation, I told him about the idea I'd been toying with all day. The long Easter weekend was coming up. "Let me try to take care of Liam this weekend."

Marc's eyebrows drew together. "But I'm working until Friday."

"I know; that's why it's perfect. My parents will be here if I need anything, but I'll do my best to take care of him myself on Thursday. Then, even though you'll be here, I'll try to do everything myself throughout the weekend. If I can do it, then we'll know it's time."

I couldn't manage Liam's diapers, so I purchased some Pull-ups. I was determined that nothing would prevent me from taking care of my son.

The first night I decided to change his diaper before bed. I smiled as I went over to him, hoping to get him to lie down. He gave me a funny little smile and ran away. He had taken his first steps a few short months after I had. It took me fifteen minutes to finally coax him onto the bed for a diaper change.

I placed my arms through the holes, and tugged the underwear-like diaper up his legs until it was securely in place. I had removed his onesie by pulling apart the snaps. As there was no chance I would get that back on him, I dressed him in a T-shirt and track pants. Oh joy! I had done it.

Because I could not go to him in the middle of the night if he called, I decided to let him sleep in the bed beside me. A couple of hours into the night, he decided he wanted to get up and play. I would coax him back down onto the bed, not giving him a chance to get out, and sing him back to sleep.

By the next morning I was exhausted, but I was determined to make it work. I was able to remove his dirty diaper and drop it on the floor in my living room, intending to throw it in the garbage later. Liam gave me a coy smile and ran down the hall naked to his bedroom. I followed him, grabbed a clean diaper from the table beside his crib, and put his new diaper on him. When I was finished, I went back out into the living room to grab his old diaper, only to find that the dog had beaten me to it. She was happily snacking on Liam's dirty diaper.

Determined to do things on my own, I managed to pick up the diaper and throw it in the garbage. Shortly after, the dog, not surprisingly, vomited all over the living room floor. *I am going to have to earn this.* I paused as I stood gazing at the mess. I could call my parents for help. *No, I can do this.* I leaned over and managed to mop up everything on the floor, chuckling at the idea of telling this story on national television.

Cienna, my unwavering supporter, came home from school and clapped her hands when she saw that I had made it through the first day. When Marc finally walked in the door, I fought the desire to hand him his son and run to my bed for rest. I had pushed and prayed through every moment, and I was able to prove it could be done.

I interviewed many candidates for the four-day-a-week position, until I met the young lady who would be our next nanny. She would be the one to help me transition from part-time mom to full-time mom once again. On her first day, she arrived with a basket full of activities and fun for the children. She quickly gained the nickname "Mary Poppins" as she came alongside me and helped me recapture the heart of my son.

Thank you, God, for that gift.

Water splashed as I dug my arm through the water, and I paused my trip down memory lane. "How many metres have I done now?"

From the far end of the pool I heard her voice, "That's seventy-five."

I am halfway there.

Enjoying my time with God, I took a deep breath and thought of my son.

The new nanny had not been with us very long when I walked across the front deck on my way to the pool. "Mama! Mama!"

I peered through the large window that spanned the length of the deck. My son was crying for me.

"You will know the day you hear him cry for you, the way your daughter does when you leave her at daycare." I had heard those words spoken so many months ago and, finally, that day had arrived. I ran inside and hugged my little boy.

Cienna became my biggest cheerleader. Every time I did something new, she would cheer me on and tell everybody. "Look, Daddy, Mommy made dinner!" she said as Marc walked through the door the first time I had accomplished the task by myself. Pasta was the easiest dish to start with, and everyone's favourite.

Each time I went to the fridge for a juice box for the kids, or I cut up vegetables or fruit on my specialized cutting board with a fixed, pivoting knife, my heart celebrated. One more step back to full-time motherhood.

"You're done 150 metres!" my physiotherapist cried from the edge of the pool.

"I'm not finished yet!" I yelled back as I pushed on. My therapists were so enthused about my swimming that they were looking into competitive clubs, but after that experience on the porch with my son, and the moments with my daughter, I knew where my time needed to go.

Thank you, God, for giving me my children back.

Nine months after the day I became ill, I retested for my driver's license. I felt confident yet nervous. Although I had practiced, I had not actually been allowed to legally drive without someone in the car. My beaming father waited for me as I exited the licensing office and said, "I did it!"

When Marc arrived home, we put both kids into the Subaru station wagon and I prepared to drive my family for the first time as a quadruple amputee. I fastened my seat belt and turned around to the children in the backseat. "Okay, kids, you are about to be driven by a woman with no hands and feet!"

As I pulled out of the driveway, I glanced over at Marc. His eyes were shining with love and pride. "You're driving!" he said as he videotaped me maneuvering the station wagon down the main street of our city, past the hospital where I had first gone when I was sick. It seemed like a lifetime ago.

"Mom, let's pull over to ask somebody if they've seen your hands," Cienna joked. I looked in the rearview mirror at the twinkling eyes of my children.

God, thank you for this first moment that I am able to drive by myself.

The most challenging activity I would encounter would be figuring out how to undo my son's car seat. Doing it up was difficult enough, but finding a way to position my stumps in the ideal spots on the clips to unhook the seat buckle turned out to be a task that would take me months to accomplish.

I hadn't had my license long when I pulled up to the house of one of Cienna's friends to pick her up and take her and Cienna to Brownies. As her mom got her settled in the car, I waited for her to take one look at me and change her mind and remove her daughter from the vehicle, but she didn't change her mind, and I drove away.

Sometimes when I'm driving down the road by myself, I gaze up at the sky and I can feel His presence. Jesus has faithfully held my hand through every moment of this long journey.

Thank you, God! You never left me. You gave me my life back.

I finished 200 metres and pulled myself out of the pool. "Give me a high stump!" I raised my arm and my therapist high-five'd me. She moved on to her next patient, but I decided to just sit on the ledge. It felt good remembering, reminiscing.

It seemed so long ago that I would lie in bed at the rehab hospital and dream about driving myself to the grocery store, or going to the drive-through to grab a coffee. Most of the people in the area have become accustomed to me, the woman with no hands pulling up to the drive-through. Some of them have even seen the media coverage of our story.

At first I was intimidated by the idea of ordering and picking up a coffee at the drive thru. I had done trial runs with my mom and our nanny before attempting a solo run.

As I sat at the kiosk waiting to speak my order, I thought, *Will my arms be long enough to reach the drink?*

When I pulled up to the window, I ensured my car was as close as possible. Warmth crawled up my face as I realized the cashier was seeing me for the first time. I dismissed her look of shock as I handed her my ten dollar bill. She made change, and I held out my arms for the coins, but she froze. *She's wondering how to hand it to me.* I took a deep breath, I had become accustomed to giving instructions.

"Put the coins in a pile and place them in between my arms." I smiled, holding my arms out. She looked even more confused.

I had an idea. "If you have an empty coffee cup, you can put my change in that." She smiled, relieved to have a solution. She placed the coins into the cup and passed it to me. She then reached over to grab the coffee and turned to put it in to my out reached arms. She hesitated again.

"Won't it burn you?" I glanced at the rearview mirror taking note of the growing line of cars behind me.

"No, my arms are tougher than that." I waved my arms at her and reached them out to quickly grab my favourite latte. Once it was between my stumps I had to concentrate with all my effort to successfully place it into my car drink holder.

My ten minute drive home was a great exercise in patience as I savoured the aroma, knowing that I could not take a sip until I had parked my car.

I still shop with Marc or the nanny or my parents, since I can't reach most of the things on the higher shelves, I can do many other things on my own.

One of the first things I attempted was to pay for groceries with my debit card. I had to shop for a purse that provided enough room for my stumps to get in and grab the card. Wallets were not something I could manage. Once I had my card between my stumps, I would slip it into the reader. Then I would enter my pin as I watched the perplexed cashier. Sometimes I could sense the discomfort of the cashier as I approached and imagine what she must be thinking. Thoughts such as, *How will she pay?* or *Will she need any help?*

At first when I went out in public, I would make a mental note of the most accessible washrooms; however, I quickly came to realize, through trial, that although a sign on the door claimed it was *accessible*, it likely wasn't for me.

At a restaurant with Marc and the kids, I proceeded to go to a washroom that I was unfamiliar with. When I closed the door, I studied the small knob inset into the door handle. *Surely if I could lock it, I could unlock it.* I placed a stump on either side of the lock and turned it. So far, so good.

I washed up and proceeded to the door, only to find that my stumps were too large to turn the lock back to let myself out. After struggling with the lock for fifteen minutes, I finally opened it. Unfortunately, I had to open it with my teeth. It was no surprise that the following week I came down with a bad cold.

Enough reminiscing. I stood up from the ledge, took a deep breath, and waved goodbye to my therapists before walking into the dressing room. Slipping my wet suit top off over my head, another memory flashed—my bra fiasco.

Most of the things I did took me at least twenty times longer than they used to, and required an immense amount of planning. A task as simple as brushing my teeth required precise movements and meticulous concentration in order for me to do it successfully. If I attempted even a relatively easy task without first devising a strategy, I would likely fail to accomplish it. I learned that one evening when I decided to put my bra on a different way than I had been doing it. I was in my bedroom getting ready to go out to dinner with Marc and the kids. They were at the front door down the hallway, waiting for me. I had always put my bra on by making sure that it was pre-fastened and sliding my legs into it, then proceeding to pull it up with my arms and wrangling the straps into place. A congenital amputee who had visited me early on had shown me this trick.

This time I tried putting the bra on over my head, but I was only able to get it as far as my underarms. Then I was stuck, a prisoner in my own bra. For fifteen minutes I lay on the bed, strategizing about how I could get my arm up under the bra to tug it down. Although my right arm was free, my left arm was trapped straight up in the air, and I was unable to reach far enough to liberate myself.

"Are you okay, honey?" The words echoed down the hallway.

Heat flooded my cheeks. "Yes!" I didn't want Marc to come in and find me looking like Houdini trapped in a failed escape attempt.

I scanned the room for something that might assist me in pulling the bra down—a door hook or anything. But I found nothing. In the end, I stretched my right arm as far as I could up and under the bra, while using my teeth to maneuver the garment back down. When I walked down the hallway, I caught a glimpse of myself in the mirror. My face was covered in red marks, and my hair was sticking straight up.

Thank you, God, for a sense of humour.

One day Marc and I were driving home from church. Turning my head to study him, I was once again reminded that he was not the same man. He had become the husband I'd always wished I had, showing me unending love and support, something that had been missing in our marriage before.

Thank you, God, for my husband.

As I bounded out of the building that housed the pool and into my car, I reflected on the truth of Job's words in the Bible, *"The Lord giveth and the Lord taketh away."* God had given to me and, yes, He had taken away. But it wasn't until He gave me back what I had lost that I was able to comprehend what a blessing it had been in the first place.

Thank you, God, for giving me back so much more than I could have ever asked for or imagined.

Epilogue

I stood in front of the large, 80s-style mirror fastened to the wall above the sink in our bathroom. The mirrored sliding doors on the bathtub behind me provided a three-hundred-and-sixty-degree view of my naked body.

My prosthetic legs looked realistic, as they had been shaped and sculpted to appear that way. They were held onto my thighs by liners—long, silver-stocking-like silicone bands that rolled up to the top of my leg, securing the human to the man-made body parts. I was a bionic woman. Led by God, medical science had rebuilt me.

My gaze travelled to the reflection of the top of my head. My hair was still very thin, but showed signs of growing back. Little baby hairs poked out at the hairline around my face and near my ears. New growth.

I still had two scars on my scalp at the back of my head from bedsores. If my hair was not parted the right way, they'd stand out and I would have exposed bald spots. At first I had wondered if I was losing my hair because of the wounds on my head. Later, I came to suspect that the loss was a side effect of the medications I was on, although that has never been confirmed.

"Hair does not grow back on scar tissue," the doctor had told me. Each time I went to the hairdresser, or someone put my hair up, I would be reminded that I had two large spots on the back of my head.

At the base of my throat is a tracheotomy scar. "It's my upper belly button," I liked to tell the kids. Around it are three more scars, to the right, to the left, and just below. I will carry this *belly button* for the rest of my life.

I thought back to the flawless body I'd had before. Except on my fingers, which I had frequently cut when chopping vegetables, there had been no scars. A smile crept up. *No need to worry about cutting my fingers now.*

As my gaze drifted around to the middle of my back, I studied two more scars. They are large indentations, bedsores caused by not being moved frequently enough when I was bedridden. Those sores had endured a few infections. Fully healed now, they continue to sit there like large craters.

My right leg is missing up to thirty-five percent of its original flesh and muscle, leaving me with a big, gaping hole. This was the spot where the necrotizing fasciitis had originally entered. The scar runs from the top of my right hip all the way to the bottom of my right stump and also sports a large crater of missing skin. That skin had been grafted back on and carries a crisscross pattern, as if chicken wire had been applied to it. I had seen the pattern on others and knew that it would also remain for the rest of my life.

The left thigh was my donor site. It has thick red stripes that will never turn back to a normal pigmentation.

None of those scars will fade.

Beautiful imperfections were woven into every scar. Each one represented a road I had taken through this journey. Each scar represented the birth of a new me. I thought back to that moment I knew I was dying. That moment in which I pleaded, *Please, God, don't take me now; I'm not ready.* God heard my plea. He gave me a second chance.

I knew the words "I'm not ready" must have meant something different to God. Those words carried a far deeper meaning to Him than they did for me at that time. Now I understood. I certainly wasn't ready. I hadn't been living for Him. I did a great job of believing in Jesus, but I certainly didn't follow Him.

My inspection moved back to my chest and then up. My eyes were the mirror to my heart. When I first came home from the hospital, my eyes continued to hold a hollow look.

"Daddy, why does Mommy sometimes look off into the distance with a strange look?" my daughter had asked.

It was the look of loss. But that look turned into one of gain as I slowly realized how blessed I was.

Now, standing in front of the mirror, examining my scarred body, broken and bent, with missing parts, all I could think was, *I have never felt more whole, more healed.*

It seemed like a lifetime ago that I sat in the bathtub and thought about taking my own life. I wanted the pain of infertility to end. Thankfully, I loved God enough not to take my own life in that moment. Yet it wasn't until I almost lost my life that I loved Jesus enough to give Him all of my life. Now that I had a second chance, I couldn't wait to see what he would do with it. I just wanted to serve Him.

Jesus told the woman who reached out to touch his robe, "Daughter, your faith has made you whole."

I felt that wholeness now in a way I had never felt it before. I had spent so much of my life struggling hard to be more to everyone, to find more, to seek more.

More had found me in a hospital room with no hands and feet, facing my darkest fears in the most inconceivable situation.

I turned away from the mirror, my heart content as I thought of Him. The scars had taken me on a long journey, but now I planted my feet upon this ground, overjoyed to be home.

As I made my way down the hallway to the rooms where I would put the children to bed, I smiled to myself. I had so many stories to tell. If this was my new life, I was like a two-year-old. I had learned to do much on my own, yet I knew who held my hand in every moment.

Although the children were not yet aware, Marc and I were about to take our family on a new, God-led adventure. We looked forward to adding several chapters to the story God had given into our care. We would be taking more leaps of faith through the "space in between."

How many new stories would I have to tell in this re-born life?

"Tell us a story," my pyjama-clad children begged from the top bunk as I entered Cienna's cotton-candy-pink room.

I sat down on the chair beside them.

Once upon a time, on the pathway of the beautiful CiLi forest, rested a little seedling.

"Tell us again why it is called CiLi Forest." Cienna wrapped an arm around Liam and pulled him closer to her.

"Because it's named after you." I crossed my legs. "Your nicknames are CiCi and LiLi, and we named the make-believe forest after you. Now let me continue ..."

The little seedling dreamt of growing tall and proud. She wanted very badly to be a pretty flower like all the other flowers in the woods, but she was surrounded by many weeds and tall trees. These weeds and trees blocked the sunlight that she needed to grow.

One of the weeds was known as the weed of "covetousness." With its large, thorny leaves, it taunted the little seedling, "Don't you want to be like the beautiful flowers in the meadow? Look how glorious they are. If you just had a little more sunlight, if you just had a little more zest, you could be like them."

The little seedling prayed, "Please, God, help me to be pretty like the flowers in the field. I want to have long, beautiful petals with bright, lovely colours." The next morning, as the little seedling felt a tiny petal growing, she was so proud. She praised her petals to all the other creatures in the forest. She quickly forgot who placed those petals upon her.

Many storms came upon the seedling. She prayed for God to help her through each one. He reached down and shielded her with His hand, but when the storm was over, she forgot Him.

In the forest, close to the little seedling, grew the "pleaser vine." This was a vine that crawled one way, then twisted around you when you least expected it. It tried to wrap itself around the little seedling. It had a voice that was sweet and cunning. "Little seedling, you must not upset the leaves that are falling upon you, and make sure you move out of the way when the squirrels come through. Little seedling, don't you want your forest friends to like you?"

The little seedling found herself moving to and fro most the day, trying not to upset any of the other creatures. At the end of day, she found that she had not grown at all, because she had spent her time trying to please others in the forest.

The worst plant of all was the "vine of unfaithfulness." This weed pricked with its thorns. It was easy for the little seedling to forget her purpose as the thorns caused pain by pricking into her stem.

A violent storm came in and pushed hard on the seedling. No matter how hard the seedling tried to grow, the storm and heavy rains would push her over.

The little seedling realized that she was not going to make it on her own. "Please, God, please let me live."

The little seedling finally understood that, without faith in God, she could not fight off the weeds and vines that taunted her. She had wanted so badly to look pretty as the other flowers did. She had searched for wholeness in others. She had placed her faith in them. And she had not grown.

God heard the prayer of the little seedling and gave her a second chance.

To this day, when you walk through CiLi Forest, you'll come across a small flower sitting just off the path. Although she is tiny, the sunlight beams upon each petal, making it sparkle with iridescent gold as if to say, "Glory to our great creator. Look at the works He has done."

And God looks down on that beautiful flower, and He smiles.

Acknowledgements

When I go to sleep at night, my heart does a little dance of joy and thanks to God who, as part of His plan, united this family.

Marc has shown unwavering support and love by ensuring I was given the time and support to write this story. It takes a strong and repentant man to be willing to expose his sins in print. I am so thankful that I get to call this man my husband.

When I received notice that *Shine On* would be published, I was with my children. They were so happy for me that they danced and cheered. I am so blessed that my cheerleader, Cienna, and my funny man, Liam, call me Mama.

I am grateful for all the love and support my parents give us every day and during the writing of this book.

I would not be published without the influence of the following: Women's Ministry Institute and the ladies involved. You grew my heart for God and subsequently a rewrite of my manuscript.

I first met Sara Davison through Ruth Coghill. Both ladies have been a breath of fresh air and have built into me as a writer. Both of these authors have been great mentors, and I am so thankful that God has united our paths.

One note of encouragement from Sylvia St. Cyr and I was furiously working to pull this book together in submission to a publishing contest.

I am so thankful to Word Alive Press and Women's Journey of Faith for giving me the opportunity to share this story.

Photo Gallery

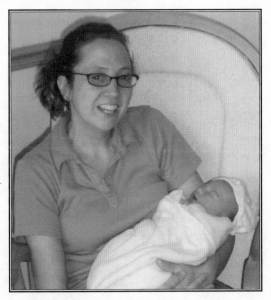

Cradling Cienna, an answered prayer

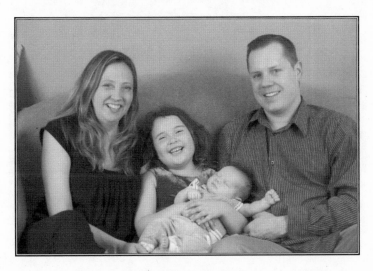

Our family is complete

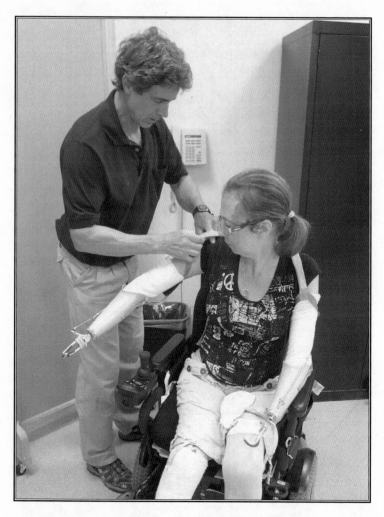

Getting fitted for new arms

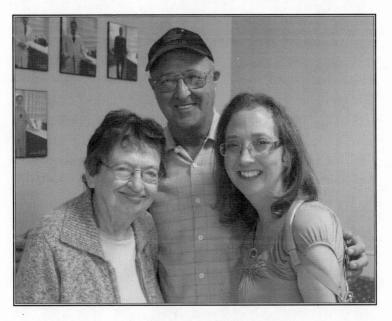

A regular visit from my Mom and Dad

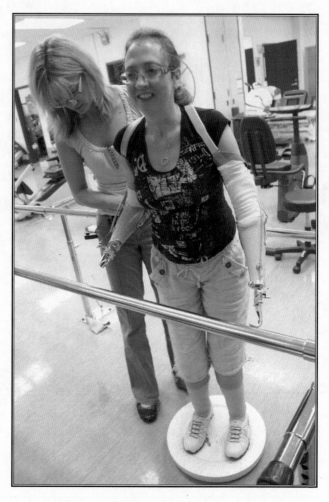

Finding a new centre of gravity

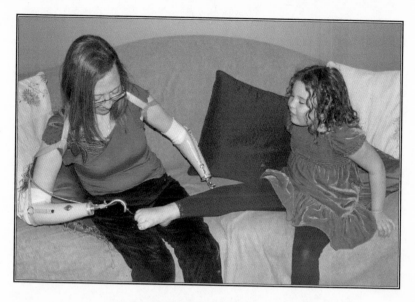

Being a "hands on" mom

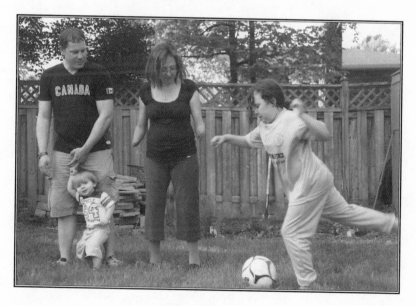

A family once again